EDWARD
JENNER

EDWARD
JENNER
THE VACCINATION VISIONARY

ROB BODDICE

Cover image courtesy of Wellcome Library, London.
pp. 6–7: James Gillray, 'The Cow-Pock – or – the Wonderful Effects of the New Inoculation!' 1802. (Wellcome Library, London)

First published 2015 as *Edward Jenner: Pocket Giants*
This edition first published 2023

The History Press
97 St George's Place, Cheltenham,
Gloucestershire, GL50 3QB
www.thehistorypress.co.uk

British Library Cataloguing in Publication Data.
A catalogue record for this book is available from the British Library.

ISBN 978 1 80399 242 6

Typesetting and origination by The History Press
Printed and bound in Great Britain by TJ Books Limited, Padstow, Cornwall.

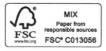

Trees for LYfe

Contents

Introduction: The Jenner Legend   9

1   Going Cuckoo   17
2   A Brief History of Smallpox   33
3   Inspiration   41
4   Hero?   53
5   Villain?   67
6   Tragedy   85
7   Legacy   99

Timeline   111
Abbreviations   113
Notes   114
Further Reading   124
Web Links   126
Acknowledgements   127
About the Author   128

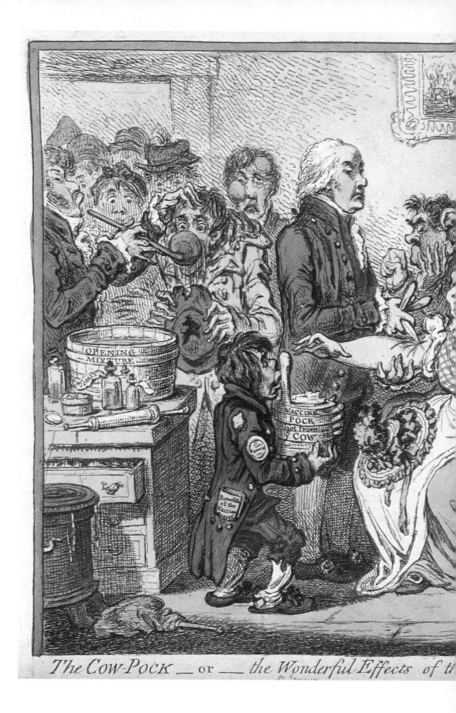

The COW-POCK __ or __ the Wonderful Effects of t[...]

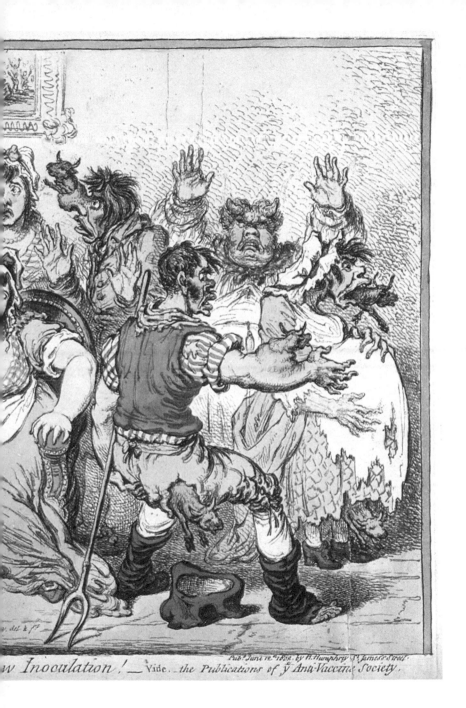

w Inoculation! — Vide the Publications of ÿ Anti-Vaccine Society.

Pubᵈ June 12 1808. by H.Humphrey Sᵗ James's Street.

Introduction

The Jenner Legend

The instrument in the hands of a gracious Providence.

John Baron, 1838[1]

Edward Jenner was the protégé, at first directly and latterly by correspondence, of John Hunter, the famous surgeon, scientist and observer. John Hunter's maxim for life, as for scientific inquiry, was 'Do, don't think'. His favourite pupil, Edward Jenner, certainly *did*.

Not all the doing was great and good. Jenner is immortalised as the man who made it possible to rid the world of one of its greatest scourges: smallpox. But along the way there was a whole host of experimental gambits, intuitive flights and spontaneous decisions. The spirit of scientific and medical investigation by induction was alive and well with Edward Jenner. Animated by scientific curiosity, without much obvious personal ambition, and driven by the energetic counsel of his mentor Hunter, Jenner shot, poked, boiled and pricked his way through a life of rural experimentation. One such experiment would provide proof of the concept for human-to-human inoculation of cowpox, which in turn provided immunity from smallpox. Jenner named the cowpox virus *Variolae vaccinae*, or smallpox of the cow, from which he derived the word 'vaccine'. But to get to this breakthrough, which came well into Jenner's middle age, we must first follow the spirit of trying things out that defined his earlier life.

To tell the life story of Jenner in this way cuts against the grain of typical narratives of his heroic life. Jenner has been – at least in the popular imagination – remembered as the saviour of more lives than any other single medical doctor. We know him as having rid the world of a terrible plague through a genius of daring experimentation, controlled trials and an indefatigable hard-nosed activism. Without these things vaccination would not have gained traction within the medical community and the global population at large. Received wisdom is that Jenner was without pecuniary interest, working for the benefit of humanity at great personal cost. He is remembered for qualities that set him apart from many of his peers. Such a rare and noble nature is the stuff of heroes.

This line of thinking has come down to us from the first memorialisation of Jenner's life, published by his friend and colleague John Baron in 1838, some fifteen years after Jenner's death. Baron was an uncritical disciple; his work was more hagiography than biography. It is filled with an expansive history of smallpox itself, and extensively documents the failings of all of Jenner's opponents. While important for some of the essential details of Jenner's life that are unobtainable elsewhere, one finds little left in the bag after shaking it free of detritus. The letters it contains are useful, but they uniformly show Jenner in the best light. What are we to make of Baron's assessment: 'Jenner stood in a position never before occupied by mortal man; having been the instrument in the hands of a gracious Providence, of influencing, in a most remarkable degree, the destinies of his species'?[2] Jenner, for Baron, was sent by God himself.

Medical historians have long been familiar with the messy and contested reality of Jenner's innovations and greatness, but there is no recent academic biography of his life in its entirety, even though much of Jenner's correspondence survives. The latest biography, by Richard Fisher, is long out of print.[3] Articles appear here and there on various aspects of Jenner's life and world, but their reception is confined to small academic audiences. Common knowledge on Jenner's life does not seem to run too deep. Considering the magnitude of Jenner's contribution to medicine, it is perhaps surprising that he continues to be known as a kind of two-dimensional saint: a saviour of humanity with a statue here and there. This reputation in not confined to Britain; it stretches from Europe to the Americas, and from the Indian subcontinent to the Far East.

How does such a hero emerge? How can such an exceptional figure rise above the clamour and change the course of history? The answer is not a mystery, but hidden in plain sight. As a country surgeon, Jenner was not so extraordinary. His was a life of parochial interest, touched and pushed in various ways by exceptional circumstances, energetic friends and sponsors, and a deep-seated awareness of the importance of public reputation. Far from being set apart from the late eighteenth-century world of medicine, gentility and Enlightenment, Jenner was immersed in it. Tucked away in rural Gloucestershire, seemingly detached from the nature-conquering endeavours of urbane men of letters, Jenner was actually steeped in Enlightenment values, borne on a wave of correspondence and personal connections in London and farther afield. Setting up a country practice to meet his material needs, Jenner was motivated to experiment by a commonly held desire to understand nature so as to *master* it. With this firmly in view, the smallpox vaccination experiments can be put into a broad context of medical, anatomical and physiological experiments that Jenner carried out at home, some of which were successful, most not. The overwhelming success of vaccination would come to define the second half of Jenner's life, but he had not planned for this. He spent his energy, with considerable chagrin, on the defence of his reputation and ended his life filled with uncertainty about his personal, professional and medical legacy.

The status of Jenner's reputation at his death and in the decades that immediately followed should make us all the more amazed that we have come to know Jenner as a hero at all. He was hounded by anti-vaccinationists in his lifetime; the anti-vaccine movement throughout the nineteenth century made serial concerted attacks on Jenner's character, his medical insight and his morality. Vaccination against smallpox would lead to riots, protests and paranoia. Vaccination was, for many, a scourge in itself, blighting children with animal or pestilential matter, and trespassing on the liberty of parents to decide what was best for their children. Anti-vaccination societies sprang up, particularly in Britain. Many prominent voices decried Jenner's work as quackery, thrust upon an ignorant and vulnerable population by government tyranny, risking the health of the poor. Jenner's allies, during his own lifetime and afterwards, fiercely defended the medical breakthrough that Jenner had made. Public opinion was polarised into Jenner-haters and Jenner-lovers. Those people who celebrated Jenner – usually prominent medical and scientific public figures – were forced to do so in unequivocal, absolutist terms, in the face of a torrent of abuse. Almost coeval with the invention of vaccination itself, therefore, arose the legend of Jenner the saviour of humanity, and the frightened naysayers of vaccination.

Edward Jenner was born in May 1749 in the village where he would come to spend most of his life, Berkeley in Gloucestershire. The son of the local vicar, Jenner was given a classical grounding for his education, first at Wotton-under-Edge and then at Cirencester. He was raised by his sisters after both of his parents died in 1754, when Edward was only 5 years old. He was probably fairly typical for a boy of his social class, making sport of the collection of nests (dormice were his special proclivity) and searching for fossils. At the age of about 14, a somewhat hypochondriacal Jenner was packed off to Sodbury near Bristol, where he became apprentice to Mr Ludlow, a local surgeon. There is little record of Jenner's time spent learning the ropes of surgery, but he clearly became competent enough to attract the attention of the London elite. In 1770, a keen 21-year-old, Jenner moved to London to work under John Hunter, residing with his family for two years and, according to Baron, becoming his 'favourite pupil'.[4] Hunter at that time was surgeon at St George's Hospital in Tooting, while also running a menagerie at Brompton for the purposes of scientific experimentation and observation. Hunter's combined interests would soon become Jenner's. There was love between the two men, in the manner of eighteenth-century relationships that were based on fellow feeling and frank exchange. But Jenner could not get on with London – he would come to have a deep resentment for it – and returned to take up his practice in Gloucestershire, dividing his time between Berkeley, his ancestral home, and Cheltenham. While Hunter may have allowed his pupil to leave, he would not leave him alone.

1

Going Cuckoo

But why think, why not try?

John Hunter, 1775[5]

The popularity of natural historical observation in England reached a peak with the publication of Gilbert White's *The Natural History of Selborne* in 1789. Jenner tapped into the popular mood, and assured himself a place of honour among scientific minds, by going cuckoo in 1788. In that year he finally published his 'Observations on the Natural History of the Cuckoo' in the *Philosophical Transactions of the Royal Society*, after more than a decade of thinking about it. The article capped years of ad hoc research in which Jenner observed, shot, collected, dissected and prepared. It is easy, perhaps, for the contemporary reader to see in Jenner's rambling and scrambling among the hedgerows, looking for birds' nests, a mark of amiable eccentricity. Yet Jenner was of a piece with many of his peers, who sought to explain the natural history of the phenomena around them by collecting, and often by killing, what they saw. Not only was his treatise accurate scientifically – it was the first to fully explain what happened to the 'siblings' of cuckoo chicks and why – it also tapped a rich vein of general interest.[6] Jenner was a man of the moment.

The cuckoo research did not come out of nowhere. Jenner was Hunter's country collector, doing experiments at his bidding and sending all manner of materials to London. Hunter wanted salmon, eels and cuckoos, and had an insatiable appetite for hedgehogs. Hunter once wrote to explain an experiment involving living bats, 'if you catch any'.[7] The 'if' was, undoubtedly, an imperative. Between them, they materially accelerated the disappearance of the bustard from England, its rareness even in the 1780s making Hunter all the more desirous of having one killed and sent. Jenner's roaming of the countryside on his way to the homes of patients provided the ideal opportunity to fill his bags. His spoils went by the new mail coach service, which started in 1784 between Bristol and London, via Bath (and which must have exercised a high degree of tolerance with Jenner's parcels). Mostly, Jenner's preparations were already dead, but sometimes they were sent to Hunter alive. As early as 1773, Hunter commissioned Jenner to provide him observations on cuckoos and on the breeding of toads, congratulating him at the same time for his success with parsnips. Within days, Jenner sent him a cuckoo's stomach by mail. Hunter demanded more, telling Jenner to start meddling with cuckoo eggs, placing them in different nests and keeping an account of his observations.

The research was anything but disciplined. Jenner, on his rounds, would stop to observe, shoot and collect. In his mid-twenties, Jenner was much more concerned with hedgehogs than with cuckoos, trying to find out (again at Hunter's behest) what happened to their temperature at different times of year. Jenner's work room at home must have been a forbidding place, as he beheaded and dissected one hedgehog after another; then cuckoos, rooks, swifts, martins, and later dogs, and the organs of cows, pigs, and, occasionally, people. Jenner was particularly interested in the sexual habits of various animals, and he carefully measured the size of the testes of many birds at different points in the season. Hunter set him about sexing eels.

Such enthusiasm for experimentation was not untypical for a young man of science, filled with Enlightenment principles. There were no ethical quandaries; only the pursuit of knowledge. This drive would come to be essential to the development of the vaccine, which employed children as Jenner's experimental subjects. Jenner's attitude towards the natural world was directed, shaped and commanded by Hunter. Any tendency to intellectual speculation was soon eliminated in favour of more practical methods. In a letter of 1775, Hunter made this perfectly clear:

> I thank you for your Exp.t on the Hedge Hog; but why do you ask me a question, by the way of solving it. I think your solution is just; but why think, why not try the Exp.t Repeat all the Exp.t upon the Hedge Hog as soon as you receive this, and they will give you the solution.[8]

Jenner's cuckoo research gives an indication of how his experimental instinct was developing; in particular, his determination to gather certain proof. Most of his observations were of cuckoos in the nests of hedge sparrows, but he also documented cuckoos being fed by other species. On one occasion he had the opportunity of seeing a cuckoo chick being fed by titlarks (pipits), which was a somewhat rare occurrence: 'I saw the old birds feed it repeatedly, and, to satisfy myself that they were really Titlarks, shot them both, and found them to be so.'[9]

There ended the vagaries of speculation, and also lives of the titlarks, and probably that of the cuckoo as well. We might now recoil from such matter-of-fact killing, but Jenner's time was not ours. Nature was then thought to be at the disposal of man, who had been nominated 'Lord of the Creation' by God. Creatures were placed on earth for the amusement and education of men, and to kill an animal for the sake of widening the scope of human knowledge was not a moral concern, but a scientific obligation. This outlook could take a local naturalist to extraordinary lengths. Perhaps the peak of Jenner's willingness to do Hunter's bidding concerned the acquisition of a porpoise. Hunter wanted one 'for either Love or Money'. In early 1777, Jenner was alerted to a female porpoise – actually it was a bottle-nosed dolphin – swimming up the Severn with a calf. He shot both, and must have recruited many people to haul the carcases out of the river. Jenner's account of this event, which he still recalled over forty years later, has a sensory quality and is filled with a kind of awe, but no sense of remorse or disgust. We might judge this harshly, but modern Western ethics and the sentiments that underlie them were not part of the emotional repertoire of the eighteenth century.

Hunter wanted the mammal 'coarsely stripp'd & the bones put into a casket and sent', which evidently happened, since it now resides in the Hunterian Museum at the Royal College of Surgeons in London. The calf was to be preserved whole if not too large. Almost giddy with excitement, Hunter was eager for Jenner to taste the porpoise's milk, telling him exactly where to find the nipples. Hunter later asked him if the milk was sweet, imploring him to preserve some if he could. Even in 1819 Jenner could recall that the 'milk was like that of the Alderney Cow'. Hunter wanted the breasts, the kidneys, the stomach and a piece of the intestines sent intact. All this Jenner did, bloodied to the elbows and relishing the chance to examine and dissect what he described as 'very wonderful animals – they seem to be the human beings of the Ocean & wherever nature could humanize them compatibly with progressive motion & their apparatus for taking their food, she does it'.[10] Notwithstanding the high place in nature accorded this class of animals, Jenner and Hunter were perfectly in accord with their era's Enlightenment ideals of mastery over nature. To skeletonise a 'whale' was a major achievement.

Throughout the dolphin episode Hunter continually pressed Jenner to get on with the cuckoo work, but Jenner was about to experience a bump in the road that would slow his progress. For several months in 1778 the correspondence between the two men dried up, specifically after Hunter wrote to Jenner in July that he had heard about Jenner's marriage to 'a young Lady with a considerable fortune'.[11] Hunter had hoped it was true, but alas Jenner was experiencing heartbreak. We do not know the details of the object of Jenner's affections or the reasons for his love remaining unrequited, but at the end of September Jenner finally told Hunter of his disappointment. Hunter's response is perhaps the best example of the nature of their relationship, which was at once tender and distant, friendly but clearly stratified. The mentor wrote to his disciple:

> I own I was at a loss to account for your silence, and I am sorry at the cause. I can easily conceive how you must feel, for you have two passions to cope with viz that of being disappointed in love and that of being deserted, but both will wear out, perhaps the first soonest. I own I was glad, when I heard that you was married to a woman of fortune; 'but let her go never mind her'. I shall employ you with Hedge Hogs.[12]

According to Baron, being occupied with hedgehogs was not an effective tonic, and Jenner suffered for some years over his loss. He wrote to his oldest local friend, Edward Gardner, some five years later, complaining of 'constant fatigue', not only of body, but also of mind. 'Still the same dead weight hangs upon my heart', he complained, describing a 'stream of unhappiness' that seemed 'inexhaustible'.[13] If Jenner was inconsolable,

Hunter was insatiable, demanding eels, hedgehogs and, relentlessly, cuckoos.

In the process of working out the peculiar life course of the cuckoo, Jenner had cause to kill a great number of them. Hunter in particular pressed his protégé to mail them to London, in various states. Through such work, Jenner refined his skills in making anatomical displays, many of which were of cuckoos. Some of his avian preparations are to be found among the prized possessions of the Hunterian Museum. Hunter thanked Jenner for sending him a cuckoo's stomach. He also wanted cuckoos' eggs and nests – a nest with an egg, a nest with a young cuckoo, and a nest with an old cuckoo (as well as crows' nests and magpies' nests). Killing females at various points in the season, Jenner was able to dissect them and display them so as to demonstrate the cuckoo's prodigious egg-laying capacities:

> That the Cuckoo actually lays a great number of eggs, dissection seems to prove very decisively. Upon a comparison I had an opportunity of making between the ovarium, or racemus vitellorum, of a female Cuckoo, killed just as she had begun to lay, and of a pullet killed in the same state, no essential difference appeared … The appearance of one killed on the third of July was very different. In this I could distinctly trace a great number of the membranes which had discharged yokes into the oviduct; and one of them appeared as if it had parted with a yolk the preceding day.[14]

This morbid anatomy was part of Jenner's proof. The cuckoo did not stay in England for long enough to rear its own young. By laying its eggs in other birds' nests, it gained the capacity for the continuous production of eggs, just as with domesticated chickens whose eggs are collected daily. In Jenner's estimation, nature had found a way for the cuckoo, briefly passing through English shores, to produce a great progeny.

Jenner killed and dissected the fauna about him yet also revered nature as an expression of God's creation. There is no contradiction in this, even though it might be difficult for us to comprehend. Jenner was Romantic as were the times (though his poetry, of which much survives, leaves something to be desired). Death was part of nature. Jenner saw the object of his study, the young cuckoo, set about killing the other birds in the nest, designed by nature to eliminate all competition. In his paper for the Royal Society, Jenner commented on the balance in the natural order of things:

> nature permits the young Cuckoo to make this great waste, yet the animals thus destroyed are not thrown away or rendered useless. At the season when this happens, great numbers of tender quadrupeds and reptiles are seeking provision; and if they find the callow nestlings which have fallen victims to the young Cuckoo, they are furnished with food well adapted to their peculiar state.[15]

In short, nature put everything in its place, for divine reasons. It was man's place to seek to understand nature, the better to revere it. To kill and contrive with nature went hand in hand with curing ailments and mastering the art of survival.

Hunter's sponsorship of Jenner's cuckoo work cannot be underrated. Without Hunter's repeated requests and guidance, Jenner probably would not have set about his systematic research. The final paper was sufficient to gain Jenner his entry into the Royal Society, becoming a fellow in early 1789. The letters FRS after a name carried a great weight of prestige and respectability, elevating the reputation of the bearer to a special rank of the medical and scientific elite. Nevertheless, Jenner would always remain on the fringes of the medical and surgical establishments. He did become a founder member, with Alexander Marcet and others, of the Medical and Chirurgical Society of London (1805), which would gradually evolve into the Royal Society of Medicine.[16] At the time, however, it was a breakaway group from the Medical Society of London, and was not significant until later. Here we find a peculiar conflict in Jenner's character: he was clearly possessed of a significant ambition and a need for recognition, but this need was balanced by a clear preference for the hedgerows of Gloucestershire, wherein lay his objects of study. Jenner felt the pull of London life and resisted. If he were to have fame, it would be chiefly by correspondence; if he were to have fortune, it would be made from his rural base.

Fortune would be some time in coming. Jenner was comfortably off, but needed to work for a living. Chasing after cuckoos and corralling hedgehogs were vocational pursuits, but these activities took place between the professional activities of meeting the needs of a fairly widespread Gloucestershire community as doctor and surgeon. He acquired his MD from St Andrews only in 1792, but this was merely to add formal title to the practical knowledge and skill he had long possessed. Of Jenner's medical rounds we know comparatively little, but for twenty-five years his activities as country surgeon would have taken up the majority of his time. Even after he became world renowned he tried to make time for his rounds. A few diaries of medical appointments, prescriptions and accounts owing survive, showing that Jenner covered many miles, often staying away from home overnight.[17]

The mundane activities of everyday practice were in sharp contrast to the excitement of the experimental pursuits that diverted and distracted him. Specialism, either in research or in aspects of medicine, was unknown, and Jenner – like many others – tried his hand at everything, from geology to optics, natural history to human physiology. He experimented on hounds with distemper, investigated the internal temperature of dogs, devised a new method of making emetic tartar and theorised about the mysteries of the migration of birds.[18] The years at the turn of the nineteenth century were the heyday of the amateur generalist.

When the Montgolfier brothers successfully launched their balloon in 1783, Jenner was eager to replicate the event for the local community. Around 1785, Jenner filled his own patched silk construction with hydrogen, testing it at first indoors in the hall of Berkeley Castle. There followed a public exhibition in which the balloon took flight, carrying a verse penned by Jenner, before descending and being refilled at a place called Kingscote, where it is reputed by some that Jenner met the woman who would become his wife, Catharine Kingscote. Baron notes that Catharine had been 'an invalid for a considerable time before her marriage', and was never in good health, so it is likely that her weak condition served as justification for Jenner's repeated visits.[19] He married shortly before he became a Fellow of the Royal Society, making the late 1780s landmark years in the life of a man who might, at that point, have considered himself set in a contented and established domestic routine. Edward and Catharine's first child, a son they named Edward, was born in late January 1789. Hunter, the obvious choice, was named godfather, a role he accepted with characteristic wit:

I wish you Joy, it never rains but it pours. Rather than the brat should not be a Christian I will stand godfather. For I should be unhappy if the poor little thing should go to the Devil because I would not stand Godfather. I hope Mrs Jenner is well and that you begin to look grave now you are a father.[20]

Jenner marked the letter 'Poor Edward!' – Hunter was hardly an exemplar of spiritual orthodoxy – but Edward Senior was clearly overjoyed by his new family, which now, at least spiritually, extended to Hunter.

Hunter himself, along with the urbane world of science and letters, remained at a distance. There were others, however, who roamed the countryside tending to patients and who wanted outlets to develop and share their interests. Jenner helped to establish the Gloucester Medical Society, comprising many of his friends and colleagues. The society provided a congenial forum for the presentation of private research, which helped formalise the exercises in scientific curiosity that filled Jenner's spare time. Here he put forward some work he had carried out on the human heart and the effects of obstructions within its cavities. His manuscript on *Angina pectoris* is preserved in the minute book of the society's transactions, showing that Jenner not only treated and observed patients with heart problems but also occasionally managed to acquire their bodies for post-mortem anatomical investigations.[21] Jenner is generally credited with advancing modern knowledge on angina, though he gained little fame in this regard.[22] Studying the ossification of the arteries and noting their symptomatic presentation, Jenner became concerned that his mentor Hunter was suffering from precisely this complaint, and this held him back. The alarming diagnosis itself might have been too much for Hunter's heart to bear. If Jenner had published, Hunter might have perished. In the end, the stress of a fierce argument brought on Hunter's heart attack and death in 1793. An examination of his heart proved Jenner's theory, but this was cold comfort. Jenner's experimental impetus, from then on, had to come from himself.

2

A Brief History of Smallpox

The speckled monster.

Edward Jenner, 1807[23]

The virtue of the vaccine for which Jenner was to achieve fame was that it provided protection against smallpox without risk, either of serious infection or of contagion. *Variolae vaccinae*, or cowpox, was only a mild discomfort to those who received it, with the promise of immunity from a much worse disease. If we are to understand the magnitude of Jenner's intervention in the medical history of smallpox, and if we are to grasp the extent to which his experimental innovations and tireless campaigning changed the world, we first need to appreciate the severity and deadliness of smallpox and the history of previous attempts to control the disease.

Many theories have abounded about the origins of smallpox, but the latest research suggests that it has ancient origins, beginning in East Asia, spreading through the Middle East and India, and from there to Africa. *Variola major*, the most virulent strain of smallpox that would blight Europe and the New World, may have first appeared in epidemic form in China as late as AD 400, speculations about Egyptian pharaohs and Athenian plagues notwithstanding. It is often given as the cause of the Antonine Plague, brought back from the Near East to the Roman Empire, which raged from AD 165 to 180 and killed more than 5 million people. The precise date of the arrival of smallpox in the European sphere is perhaps of little consequence; what we do know is that it ravaged European populations from the Middle Ages onwards and was spread to the New World by Spanish and Portuguese expansion. Whether or not it was instrumental in the fall of Rome, we know for sure that the Spanish Empire was built upon the introduction of the disease, practically annihilating native populations in South America. By the eighteenth century, according to one estimate, smallpox claimed 400,000 lives annually in Europe, and a third of all survivors were blinded by the disease.[24] Survival was not necessarily a blessing. The characteristic pustules of smallpox that covered the face and body often left devastating scarring that marked victims for life. Since almost everyone could count on a dose of smallpox at some point in their lives, some degree of disfigurement was an everyday inevitability.

In the early eighteenth century, European travellers to Asia Minor began to hear tales of local methods, not so much of smallpox prevention as of smallpox mitigation. Inoculation or variolation practices existed across Asia and were picked up by Europeans in Istanbul. The premise was simple enough: deliberately infect a person with smallpox by inserting matter from a smallpox pustule under the skin. By infecting people in this way, the smallpox disease seemed to take a fairly benign course, with only a few pustules, and provided lifelong immunity after that. It was not foolproof, and many people died from the inoculation. Moreover, once infected in this way, the carrier was fully contagious and could infect others with the deadly confluent virus, which covered the patient with blisters. Still, at that time inoculation with smallpox seemed to be the most effective way of controlling the disease, the contraction of which seemed inevitable in any case. Inoculation was famously introduced into Europe by the tireless activity of Lady Mary Wortley Montagu, who had herself been disfigured by the disease. Witnessing the practice of inoculation in Istanbul, she had it performed on her own son to good effect. After her return to England she had her daughter inoculated under the observation of court physicians in the early 1720s. Further trials were made on prisoners and orphans, all of whom survived, and the practice was given a guarantee of both safety and popularity when it was taken up by the Princess of Wales, who submitted her two daughters to be inoculated.[25]

The reality, however, was that it was neither safe nor predictable, and the popularity of variolation was countered by vehement and nervous opposition. As physicians constructed esoteric procedures around the central variolation technique in order to make money, those who could not afford the procedure were often put in harm's way. Variolation, for the most part, ensured that the patient would get off lightly with a gentle dose of the smallpox, but it also directly abetted the spread of smallpox among the population at large. Only a few practitioners understood the need for isolation after infection, with the result that epidemics were regularly fuelled by the treatment designed to prevent disaster. Nevertheless, statistical analysis carried out by self-interested parties pointed out that the mortality rate among those inoculated with smallpox was ten times lower than for those who caught smallpox in the regular way. The danger of contagion, therefore, was overlooked in favour of a clamour for the practice by those who had access to it. Under such conditions, inoculation was introduced at Boston in the New World by Mather and Boylston in 1721, causing a riotous dispute while a deadly epidemic raged. Meanwhile in Europe the practice was adopted by royal courts and attained widespread appeal. Even though 2 to 3 per cent of those inoculated actually died from smallpox, the practice was an established norm by the middle of the eighteenth century.[26] Institutionalised inoculation practices ensured that contagious matter was ever-present among the population.

The inoculation story of one Edward Jenner is perhaps as representative as any that might be plucked from this period. At the age of 8, while being educated at Wotton-under-Edge, he was subjected to the variolation experience. The preparation took six weeks, during which time he was bled (bleeding was eighteenth-century medicine's answer to most things), purged and practically starved. The rationale for this procedure, 'to sweeten the blood', left the otherwise 'ruddy' boy Jenner 'emaciated and feeble'. The recorder of these details, Thomas Fosbroke, was recalling Jenner's youth with the advantage of more than two decades of safe vaccination behind him.

The refined medical practice of the 1820s, at least as far as smallpox was concerned, made the 1750s look like the Dark Ages. Inoculation procedures were a 'barbarism of human-veterinary practice', according to Fosbroke. After the preparation, Jenner was given a dose of the disease, presumably via a lancet in the arm. He probably remained in one of the 'inoculation stables' for two weeks, with others in a similar state, before slowly being brought back to health.[27] Some have claimed that this experience set Jenner on his life course, but it seems unlikely. After all, his suffering was in the regular order of things; smallpox inoculation was a rite of passage, a necessary evil, an awful commonplace. Jenner himself would perpetuate this rite, variolating patients well into the 1790s.

3

Inspiration

But now listen to the most delightful part of my story.
Edward Jenner, 1796[28]

There has been a great deal of hand-wringing concerning to whom the honour of discovering vaccination should go. There are various claimants, the most notable perhaps being Benjamin Jesty and John Fewster. Jesty took his family to visit a cow infected with cowpox in 1774, inoculating them purposely and directly from the site of the infection. Fewster had presented a paper to the Medical Society of London called 'Cowpox and its Ability to Prevent Smallpox' in 1765. Jesty's actions, which brought him into some disrepute, were based on local knowledge that cowpox afforded immunity from the smallpox. Jenner also based his experiments effectively on farmers' gossip that those people who had naturally had cowpox tended to be immune to attempts to inoculate them with smallpox. Baron claimed that Jenner knew of this before 1770.[29] The real 'discoverers' of the prophylactic powers of cowpox – the word 'vaccine' comes the Latin word for cow – were, therefore, the rural communities of Gloucestershire and Dorset. Fewster, too, apparently made the connection after a patient told him he had had cowpox, which might account for why he could not be inoculated with smallpox. Jesty used this local knowledge and took positive action to protect his own family, but stopped there. Fewster went somewhat further, trying out the idea on the medical community, but did not pursue it. Jenner used the local knowledge and took positive action to test it, prove its efficacy, disseminate his results and promote the practice to humanity at large. Moreover, Jenner was the first to carry out a human-to-human cowpox inoculation, proving that the operation could easily be scaled up through human incubation. At first, cowpox matter had to be taken from a cow and inserted into a human arm. Once the disease 'took', new cowpox matter could be harvested from the pustule on the arm, making it much easier to 'manufacture' the vaccine. The history of science and medicine shows that discoveries need to be brought to the fore; old paradigms have to be forcefully pushed aside, and this often involves overcoming great resistance from the guardians of prevailing knowledge. In this regard, the rural population of certain parts of England, the farmer Jesty and Dr Fewster do not deserve the credit. A medical leap may begin with discovery, but it does not end with it. Edward Jenner is indisputably the man who brought the efficacy of vaccination to light, tested it, campaigned tirelessly for its adoption and faced the waves of opposition that the discovery aroused. It is because of these things that Jenner clearly pioneered the *practice* of vaccination, without which the *discovery* would have been worthless.

It is likely that Fewster and Jenner had personally conversed on the subject of vaccination. They both attended a Convivio-Medical Society at the Ship Inn in

Alveston, and Jenner was wont to talk about the possibility to anyone who would listen. He expounded on the subject of cowpox in the mid-1780s to the point, according to Baron, that his colleagues 'threatened to expel him if he continued to harass them with so unprofitable a subject'. The surgeon Everard Home, another pupil of John Hunter, testified that Jenner had pitched his ideas about cowpox inoculation to Hunter as early as 1788. The Gloucester Society, which would supersede the one in Alveston, had also certainly heard Jenner's ideas about potential new ways to prevent smallpox infection. In 1790 Jenner began writing, on the back of a minute in the society's record of transactions, on the subject of what some Gloucestershire locals called the 'pig pox', which was spreading locally at that time. At this point Jenner had not begun his smallpox experiments, but the kernel of truth was already firmly in his mind and those of his colleagues. This small manuscript fragment notes: 'It is believed that this disease acquired wither in the natural way or by inoculation, is capable of preserving the patient from the infection of the small-pox.'[30]

Jenner used the outbreak of pig pox, or swine pox, to experiment on a subject close at hand: his baby son. Edward Jr was around ten months old when Edward Sr inoculated him with swine pox.[31] Nobody was quite sure what the swine pox was, except that it was probably related to smallpox. The boy fell ill on the eighth day and erupted in pustules, which meant that the swine pox was probably smallpox after all. To test the effect, Jenner inserted true smallpox into his arms on five or six occasions, with no result. Although this seems like the most horrendous and unethical abuse, if we recall that at this time children were commonly inoculated with smallpox – effectively given a highly contagious disease – then Jenner's actions can be better understood. He would have given his son the smallpox, as he himself had been given it as a child, had there been no other option. Swine pox presented the first opportunity to try something potentially *less* harmful than common medical practice prescribed. A year and a half later Jenner again tried to give his son smallpox, and tried again another year after that. The child suffered a local infection of the skin caused by the cut, but did not show signs of smallpox. An experimental journey had begun.

Throughout Jenner's early experience as a doctor in the 1770s he was inoculating children with smallpox, but from time to time a patient did not develop the disease, despite his efforts. In two cases where the inoculation failed, he noted that the patients had recently had severe cowpox infections. He rapidly built up enough cases to make a firm theory that once a person had had cowpox, they were 'for ever after secure from the infection of the small-pox'.[32]

The experimental journey was not without confusion. In addition to the somewhat mysterious swine pox, Jenner had to reckon with a disease called 'grease', which afflicted the heels of horses. He was convinced, and would remain so for many years, that cowpox originated in this equine malady. This seemed to be of great importance to Jenner and it would cause him much trouble in later years once it was clear that there was no relation whatsoever. Since he gave this error a prominent position in his early publications on the vaccine, it detracted from the things he got right. He tried inoculating children with grease but got nowhere. His success with inoculating cowpox, which might well have led him to drop the matter of horses' heels, instead seemed to intensify the mystery in his mind. Hindsight affords us a clarity of vision unavailable in the moment. Regardless, Jenner's experimentation did yield exciting results.

In July 1796 Jenner wrote to Gardner to announce his success. A woman called Sarah Nelmes had picked up the cowpox naturally, from a cow called Blossom. He sketched her affliction for his first publication, thereby immortalising her disease. From the pustules on her hands he inoculated an 8 year-old boy, James Phipps, on 14 May 1796. He was thrilled to report that 'I have at length accomplished what I have been so long waiting for, the passing of the vaccine Virus from one human Being to another by the ordinary mode of Inoculation.' With this, Jenner went further than anyone else who might have had a claim to have originated the idea of cowpox as preventative of smallpox. He then took a distinctly modern step even further: 'But now listen to the most delightful part of my story. The Boy has since been inoculated for the Small pox which as I ventured to predict produc'd no effect.' Just as with his inoculations of his son with swine pox, Jenner deliberately attempted to give Phipps smallpox. It was the only method available to test the efficacy of the vaccine virus. Again, our ethical misgivings have to be mitigated by the knowledge that Phipps would have been inoculated with smallpox in any case. He was Jenner's guinea pig, but he was also the first person to be protected against the smallpox with something other than smallpox itself. Success led Jenner to pursue his experiments 'with redoubled ardor'.[33]

It was among Jenner's principles to share. He did not think of the money to be made from his research. He could not abide the thought of setting up in practice in London (he later tried it and hated it). He sought, first and foremost, to spread the word. A formal channel for publication was eschewed in favour of a private printing, putting the onus on Jenner himself to drive awareness and distribution of the vaccine virus. The work, snappily titled *An Inquiry into the Causes and Effects of the Variolae Vaccinae: A Disease Discovered in Some of the Western Counties of England, Particularly Gloucestershire, and Known by the Name of the Cow Pox*, was published in 1798. Jenner's thesis was infectious: his disease treatise spread rapidly. Perhaps the most important observation in it, beyond the prophylactic powers of cowpox, was the fact that this disease was not contagious. For the duration of his time under Jenner's experimental gaze, the boy Phipps had slept in a bed with two other children who had survived their close proximity without contracting either smallpox or cowpox. Such a powerful new weapon against the smallpox was a hammer blow for the disease, but also for the widespread and lucrative practice of smallpox inoculation. A murmur ran through the medical community, at once of excitement and of fear. Jenner's *Inquiry* might prove a bulwark against infection and, worryingly, cost physicians an important part of their income by depriving them of inoculation. Jenner might become a medical hero, but in the first instance he was more likely considered an economic villain.

While in London putting the finishing touches to the *Inquiry*, Jenner more or less failed to persuade anybody of the importance of his breakthrough. He had taken vaccine lymph with him, but couldn't find a London guinea pig. It would eventually be used by Henry Cline, who became Jenner's first convert. The pamphlet contained many potential difficulties for any practitioner wishing to take up the practice. The biggest of these seemed to be the lack of precision about how to identify cowpox, since there seemed to be at least two types, of which only one had the desired effect. Furthermore, Jenner was aware that for human-to-human transfer of the virus to work properly the disease had to be captured at just the right moment, before putrefaction set in. Though the Jennerian method of vaccination was remarkably well developed from the beginning, clarification was absolutely necessary, spelling out the differences between 'true' and 'spurious' cowpox, and clearly defining when the virus pustule on the arm was fit for harvesting. Thus followed Jenner's *Further Observations on the Variolæ Vaccinæ, or Cow-Pox* in 1799 and his *A Continuation of Facts and Observations Relative to the Variolæ Vaccinæ* in 1800.

The urgency of these publications was acute. Jenner's discovery was put at risk by the catastrophic blunder of some of his earliest followers. Cowpox had been found in London, and it had come to the attention of Dr William Woodville of the London Smallpox and Inoculation Hospitals. Together with George Pearson, one of Jenner's early opportunist fans, and other interested parties, they visited the infected cows while consulting Jenner's *Inquiry*. From the matter collected from these cows, and from further matter collected by Pearson at another London dairy, the first large-scale trial of vaccination began. Unfortunately, much of the trial took place within the smallpox hospital, among patients who had or were already exposed to smallpox. The results were different to what Jenner had seen before, with eruptions that looked a lot like smallpox. The cross-contamination of cowpox and smallpox matter was an early disaster for vaccination. Pearson and Woodville were particularly industrious in harvesting and broadcasting this contaminated material, sending threads dipped in the contaminated lymph through the post to recipients who would then infect their patients with smallpox. Since the principle of Jenner's method was that vaccination could be carried on from arm to arm, this disaster risked Jenner's credibility. His own results looked different to those of medical men who started to celebrate him. Malpractice followed practice with an alarming alacrity. New vaccine enthusiasts were in fact distributing smallpox, tainting the name of vaccination with quackery. Jenner was eventually drawn to denounce Pearson and Woodville in public, in an action that would damage what had initially promised to be collegial friendships: 'where *variolous pustules* have appeared, *variolous matter* has occasioned them.'[34] The sous chefs had spoilt the broth.

Another intractable problem was indicated by Jenner himself, and for the first years of vaccination he risked losing control of the discourse he had initiated. In his original *Inquiry* on the vaccine, Jenner had stated that smallpox itself was the result of an association with animals not intended for human company. It was a disease of civilisation, typified by the 'Wolf, disarm'd of ferocity ... now pillow'd in the Lady's lap'.[35] This transgression – of communing with rather than dominating nature – had given rise to disease. His solution was to embody the substance of an animal in order to be protected from brutish disease. The idea of sullying human blood with diseased matter from the teat of a cow was abhorrent to many and sent a shock wave of disgust through polite society. Was the price for protection against smallpox the ready acceptance of becoming bovine? This was the tenor of the objection of Jenner's chief opponent, Dr Benjamin Moseley, who linked this '*bestial* humour' to a bovine form of syphilis, civilisation's other great scourge.[36]

The fear was immortalised and ridiculed by the most celebrated caricaturist of the age, James Gillray, in 1802. The 'Wonderful Effects of the New Inoculation' (see pp. 6–7) would lend Jenner's opponents plenty of inspiration in the coming years, but the attention of Gillray is indicative of success rather than failure. Jenner had caught the public's attention: his name spread by the chattering classes, his fame secure enough to withstand the onslaught of satirists. It had perhaps been so since early in the year 1800, when Jenner had been summoned to an audience with George III. Finding a favourable reception at court, Jenner dedicated the second edition of his *Inquiry* to the king.

4

Hero?

Parliament last night voted me the sum of £20,000
for making public my Vaccine Discovery.

Edward Jenner, 1807[37]

There are two ways to tell the story of vaccination in its first two decades of use. The first is as a story of success, with Jenner as its hero; the second is as a story of personal and political strife, medical quackery and jealousy, with Jenner as the villain. While it is certainly true that the first of these two narratives now stands out as the 'correct' one, this was far from clear, at least in England, in Jenner's lifetime and in the decades immediately after his death. A great many medical luminaries pronounced Jenner's innovation a medical miracle, with a conviction bordering on the religious, and vaccination spread around the globe at a speed that seems startling even now. But at the same time, large portions of the medical elite and of the general public, especially at home, repeatedly and loudly declaimed against Jenner and his methods, denigrating vaccination and defaming the man. The reality – both in terms of Jenner's life and the medical merits of vaccination – is an admixture of the two narratives. This and the next chapters explore each side of the story, from which Edward Jenner emerges as a complex character, bearing the weight of an extraordinary discovery and an even greater responsibility to implement it successfully.

Jenner certainly accrued enough baubles and rewards in his own lifetime to think himself a success. Baron dutifully records them all at the very close of his biography, taking up eight pages. Among the more significant are honorary doctorates from Harvard in 1803 and Oxford in 1813; awards of the Freedom of the City of London, Dublin, Edinburgh, Glasgow, the Borough of Liverpool and the Burgh of Kirkaldy; honorary memberships or associations with the most prestigious medical societies in France, Prussia, Bavaria, Spain, Russia, Sweden, the USA, Scotland and England; and medals struck in London, Berlin, Bologna and Paris (the Napoleon Medal). In addition, Jenner was awarded a total of £30,000 by the British Parliament in two grants, in recognition of his achievements and as recompense for his personal expenses. According to one metric that assesses the 'economic status value' of this income, it would be something over £30 million in today's money. In 1814 he had an audience with Tsar Alexander I of Russia, who congratulated him on the success of vaccination in Russia. In 1821 he was appointed physician-extraordinary to King George IV.[38] Is this not truly the curriculum vitae of a hero?

Aside from the tokens of prestige, there is plenty of other evidence that Jenner actively sought to disseminate his discovery to all peoples of all places. He had directly influenced the introduction of vaccination to North America, in 1798, having sent vaccine matter to his friend John Clinch, who had taken up a ministry in

Newfoundland. Benjamin Waterhouse, who performed the first vaccination in the United States in 1800, also received his vaccine matter from a source that originated with Jenner himself. Jenner later sent his work on vaccination to North America in the hands of Colonel Francis Gore, with the explicit instruction to reach the indigenous populations of Upper Canada. In 1807 a presentation was made to the chiefs of the Five Nations at Fort George, at which they accepted the Jennerian message and in turn sent Jenner a Wampum belt to acknowledge his precious gift. Jenner treasured it.[39] His typical course of intervention was, however, much more direct. Vaccine lymph could be preserved by various techniques, and was therefore fit for export, either between slides of glass, on ivory points made for the purpose, or even on bits of thread. Jenner sent supplies of his own stock of cowpox lymph around the world, where it worked in the same manner as a yeasty friendship cake. Once the lymph was reanimated by the addition of water, it could be injected into a host (usually a child), from which a fresh supply would arise on the arm sufficient to vaccinate a number of others. Within weeks, a seemingly endless supply of lymph taken directly from the arms of children would be available. There were no ethical qualms. As Jenner pointed out to Hugh Scott, sixth Baron Polwarth, when he sent him threads of cowpox virus: 'the matter may be generated for further use if it should fail to infect in the first instance. In every Town or Village some poor Children may be found for this purpose.'[40]

Jenner had no scruples about the social class, race or gender of his correspondents. He sent lymph to men and women of all nations and stations, and saw nothing wrong with non-medical people performing vaccinations in their locales, providing they followed his precise instructions. He sent lymph on ivory points to Lady Brome in Suffolk, and glass slides, string and ivory points to a correspondent in Leipzig, to be sure that at least one out of three would survive. Ivory points were sent aboard ships across the Atlantic and to numerous correspondents in Europe. Cowpox was occasionally found to be naturally occurring in other parts of the world, but a great many of the early vaccinations were made with lymph that had originally been collected by Jenner himself.[41]

Jenner disregarded politics too. At the time of his discovery, British relations with France were extremely unstable, and the spread of vaccination throughout Europe took place in the theatre of war. Jenner frequently lamented the comparatively low level of success in the uptake of vaccination at home, compared with the wonders it worked among enemy armies and competing empires. In 1806 Jenner received a communication from Madrid about the return of Francis Xavier Balmis, surgeon-extraordinary to King Charles IV of Spain, after a world voyage of nearly three years. Balmis had, with royal approval, undertaken the voyage in order to introduce vaccination throughout the Spanish Empire, both its South American and Asian colonies, and succeeded also in persuading Portuguese settlements to take it up, as well as introducing vaccination in China. Spain was, at that moment, an ally of France. The Bourbon line in Spain would fall shortly afterwards, with Napoleon positioning his brother on the throne. Nevertheless, Jenner was thrilled. 'What a glorious enterprize!' he wrote to Mr Phillips, founder and proprietor of the influential *Monthly Magazine*, continuing, '*I* have made peace with Spain, and quite adore her philanthropic monarch'.[42]

This was far from Jenner's only connection with the enemy. Napoleon had honoured Jenner with a medal for his discovery because of the profound benefit it had bestowed on the health of Napoleon's armies and on the population of the French Empire in general. Jenner's *Inquiry* had found its way to Geneva, Hanover and Vienna as early as 1799, and was soon being translated into various languages. The French translation was a hit in Paris in 1800, and vaccination was soon underway. A Spanish translation was ready by 1801, and the practice rapidly spread.[43] Baron collated the data from a report of the Committee of Vaccination in France in order to show that millions of individuals had been vaccinated in a short period. The number of deaths per year had reduced from around 150,000 to only 8,500, which meant that more than 140,000 children per year were being preserved by Jenner's method and as a direct result of the influence of Jenner's *Inquiry*.[44] The numbers may not have been entirely accurate, but they were enormously significant.

Jenner, therefore, was a hero in France, and he used his fame and glory to good effect. Jenner was no Bonapartist, but he wasn't shy of deference in aid of a worthy cause. On at least three occasions Jenner petitioned to have compatriots released from captivity in various parts of France. In September 1803 he petitioned a French physician to intervene in the safe return of some friends of friends, in return for the obligation he had conferred 'on every nation on the Earth by the discovery I had made & communicated'.[45] Then in 1805 he directly appealed to Napoleon himself, writing to the self-crowned emperor for the release of two English non-combatants caught up in the maelstrom of war, at Nancy and Geneva respectively. Again, vaccination's success seemed to mean that the world owed Jenner a favour:

> Sire,
>
> Having by the blessing of Providence made a discovery of which all nations acknowledge the beneficial effects, I presume upon that plea alone, with great deference, to request a favour from your Imperial Majesty, who early appreciated the importance of vaccination and encouraged its propagation ... Should your Imperial Majesty be pleased to listen to the prayer of my petition, you will impress my mind with sentiments of gratitude never to be effaced.[46]

According to Baron, Napoleon was reminded of Jenner's fame by Josephine and exclaimed that nothing could be refused to that man. The tale may be apocryphal, but the men were duly released. Jenner managed, remarkably, to be the saviour of enemy nations, the hero in the eyes of enemy leaders, and yet fulfil a duty of patriotism at home. On one occasion he even petitioned the British government, at first unsuccessfully, to release a French officer, the brother of a French physician friend. Annoyed at the snub, he instead arranged a prisoner swap for an English officer, again managing to get a petition via his contacts into the hands of Napoleon.[47] To his sister he put forward his private sentiments, hoping anyone capable of handling a weapon would volunteer to stand in the way of Napoleon's armies:

> The Invasion I know is not a popular idea with many of the greatest Generals in France, but no entreaties can make Bonaparte relinquish it. But this aspiring Mortal, who has dazzled the eyes of the World by his Feats in War, has nevertheless been for some time deprived of the use of his right reason. Heaven restore it to him, or in pity to suffering humanity remove him from this Planet, which he has thrown into such a horrid state of disorder & Confusion.[48]

Then again, he told Thomas Pruen some years later that he would 'much rather see our Island in the possession of the French, than in the hands of our own Rabble. That would be terrible indeed.'[49]

That sentiment was born of an enduring feeling of unease at the ignorance of people at home who feared vaccination. Nevertheless, the esteem in which Jenner was held abroad was generally matched at home. The practices and institutions Jenner set in motion were associated with the fame and glory of his name. As with his earlier minor successes, such as the emetic tartar, Jenner had refused to patent the vaccine and had set about immediately making his discoveries public. This was in contrast to the inoculation practices of others whose private practices had flourished on the back of proprietary quackery. He had a large volume of correspondence to deal with, a deeply felt but somewhat resented obligation to be in London, and little time to look after his own livelihood. A principal result of his acts of benevolence was that, fairly soon after his *Inquiry* was published, Jenner was hard up. He told John Clinch that he was 'some thousands out of Pocket by the necessity ... of living so much in London & throwing myself out of the way of business that brought me in a good income'.[50]

The solution to this was to petition Parliament for *post hoc* payment, based on his contribution to the well-being of humanity. It is not a model for research that many academics would care to endorse today! The petition was introduced in 1802 and the committee that discussed its merits firmly decided in Jenner's favour. There was even a declaration of optimism in accord with Jenner's own ambition to 'absolutely extinguish one of the most destructive disorders by which the human race has been visited'. Jenner had swelled the written evidence, collecting testimony from around the country and beyond on the efficacy of vaccination practice. He was particularly pleased to include a report from Copenhagen that detailed the Danish king's command that soldiers, their families, sailors, students and the poor be freely vaccinated. In general the assembled parliamentarians agreed that Jenner's discovery, combined with his selflessness in publicising and practising it, was of great benefit both to the nation and to humanity at large. There was one notable dissenting voice, whom we shall meet in the following chapter. The debate, insofar as it went, concerned the extent of the financial reward due to a man who had invested his own time and money in the saving of the lives of others, thereby indirectly swelling the coffers of the Exchequer. Many claimed that Jenner might have made £10,000 a year if he had kept his methods secret or protected them by patent. In the end this was the amount of the whole award, the House being narrowly swayed by the arguments of the chancellor to reject a more sizeable show of gratitude. Being prudent with the public purse strings was the chancellor's concern, but he was satisfied that the honour done to Jenner in Parliament was, in itself, 'a reward that would last for ever'. As it turned out, the amount was considered wholly inadequate by many of Jenner's allies, who publicly said as much.[51]

Despite this, vaccination seemed to be a waning practice. As is so often the case with medical and scientific innovation, there was a lack of effective communication in relaying the benefits to the public at large; instead, the public was subjected to literature that was more easily digested, excerpted and sloganised. Jenner had the weight of educated opinion behind him, but this was not sufficient to shift the prejudice wrought by anti-vaccinationist pamphleteers. Rallying to the cause, in 1806 Lord Henry Petty moved in Parliament that the Royal College of Physicians thoroughly investigate the practice of vaccination and report back to Parliament. Jenner was thrilled, especially since it became clear that the college would be highly favourable in its report. He thought it would destroy 'all those troublesome ghosts which have so long haunted the metropolis with their *ox-faces* and dismal hootings against vaccination'. Moreover it would formally establish 'the safety & efficacy of Vaccine Inoculation'. Lord Henry Petty's ulterior motive was to confirm the backing of the medical profession for the value of vaccination to the nation and hence gain a further Parliamentary grant for Jenner. The plan worked perfectly. A committee discussed the matter of the value of a new reward for Jenner, with the result amounting to £20,000. The news just in from Madrid about the expedition of Balmis added great weight to the College of Physicians' report. Such luminaries as William Wilberforce and William Windham were unequivocal concerning the heroic merits of Jenner's discovery and his selflessness.[52] The combined sum of £30,000, together with subscriptions sent to him from various parts of a grateful India, put Jenner in a much more comfortable position.

By the time of his second award, Jenner had much stronger institutional support behind him. A group of influential men were deeply impressed by Jenner's innovation and saw a need to organise the effective and widespread, if not universal, delivery of vaccination. They had met in London in late 1802 to discuss organising an institution to look after the interests of vaccination and resolved to proceed, but they needed Jenner at its head. It was to be a 'Jennerian Institution', so as to 'pay to the author' of the benefits of vaccination the 'first and best tribute of respect and Gratitude'. Jenner, finally enjoying some relief from hardship with the first Parliamentary award, was loath to go again to London, but deeply impressed with the idea of a society in his name. The institution set out from the first explicitly to 'eradicate the greatest scourge that ever afflicted Mankind'.[53] Jenner was considered, just as Baron would later paint him, to be the instrument of Providence.

Fairly quickly the Jennerian Society, as it became known, attracted royal patronage and set up an establishment in Salisbury Square in London. It not only sought to vaccinate the public from its own premises, but also to distribute the means to vaccinate – namely the vaccine virus – to correspondents across the globe, from India to Jamaica. The committee of the Royal Jennerian were made aware of Jenner's personal costs, and directly contributed to his personal cause for remuneration from Parliament. It reported to the inquiry of the Royal College of Physicians that between February 1803 and October 1806, the Institution had carried out nearly 21,000 vaccinations and had only recorded five failures. A giant slice of proof of the efficacy of vaccination came sealed under Jenner's own name, but with the reliability of a professionally run organisation.[54]

The major problem, however, was a chronic lack of funds. With a movement underway to establish a publicly funded National Vaccine Establishment, the Royal Jennerian wound up its business in August 1809.[55] Jenner was intimately involved with the plans for the new establishment, which caused him to be in London for more than five hateful months during 1808. With the efficacy and safety of vaccination endorsed by the Royal College of Physicians and twice by Parliament, the founding of a national instrument to deliver Jenner's vision of a society free of smallpox ought to have signified the highest expression of honour and success. But the National Vaccine Establishment was to deliver not so much the well-deserved laurels as a crown of thorns. To comprehend the dishonourable cut that Jenner felt in these circumstances we must turn to the side of his character that the hagiographers tend to overlook. Although by 1807 Jenner had filled his purse with money, he had far greater concerns: reputation, reputation, reputation!

5

Villain?

They now by the most abominable falsities endeavour to ruin my private character.

Edward Jenner, 1808[56]

The first two thirds of Jenner's life had been fuelled by curiosity, but if he had striven for anything it had been domestic contentment. His quest for quietude became more ardent in the last third of his life. Yet his deep desire to be at home, out of the fray, pottering in the hedgerows, was blighted not only by the necessary business that had grown up around vaccination, but also by his own deep concern over the way he was publicly perceived. The life of a gentleman in the early nineteenth century depended on his reputation; honour was everything. Jenner was, on the whole, outside the medical institutions whose names bestowed such honour. His peripheral presence in the medical establishment made him all the more guarded about his good name, even though he had no desire to be at the centre of things.

To understand the fallout over the National Vaccine Establishment, it is necessary to return to the first stirrings of jealousy after the publication of Jenner's *Inquiry*. Almost immediately Jenner's name had been surrounded by controversy. In public his vaccine was denounced as medical nonsense, or it was appropriated by the unscrupulous, who coveted an income. The anti-vaccinationists bothered Jenner enormously, but their denunciations came from the gutter and he scrupled not to stoop so low. He thought himself above the libellous squabbles of pamphleteers, and he frequently lamented the depths to which his friend and ally John Ring sank in order to take shots at the anti-vaccinationists. Certainly, the anti-vaccine crowd was defined by its appeals to baser instincts and common fears. The works of Moseley, as well as those by the notorious 'Squirrel' (John Gale Jones) and the 'sad wicked fellow' Birch, irritated Jenner but did not move him. He thought he had placed vaccination 'on a rock, where I knew it would be immovable, before I invited the public to look at it', and as such the cranks did not wound him.[57]

On one occasion, however, Jenner was so incensed by the false characterisation of his discovery, his work and the dangerous after-effects of vaccination that he entered into the fray, albeit anonymously. The faintly ridiculous assertions of one Dr Rowley, a noted variolator, were potentially very damaging to the vaccination cause. Rowley annoyed Jenner on two principal counts: Rowley had threatened to publish 'the names of respectable gentlemen vaccinators' who had been involved in 'the many disastrous cases' if he were attacked by anonymous reviewers from the vaccine camp; second, he had produced 'evidence' of such disasters in the form of portraits of the 'Oxfaced Boy' and the 'Mange Girl'. These absurd illustrations were meant to highlight the apparent animalistic taint that vaccination could leave. It was an underhand attempt to make real the fears that

Gillray had mocked in his earlier caricature of the effects of cowpox.[58]

Jenner wanted to round on Rowley and his ilk and give them a satirical taste of their own medicine. Jenner wrote such a manuscript and showed it to Baron, but Baron insisted that Jenner never let it get to publication, since such a temperate, rational soul as Jenner should not sink so low. Baron thought that a 'serious reply to such disgusting observations as characterised their productions would indeed have been quite unworthy' of Jenner, but he conceded that Jenner thought that 'ridicule was a weapon that might be fairly and effectually wielded'. The manuscript was styled, according to Baron, as a 'letter to one of the chief anti-vaccinists', filled with 'genuine wit and polished irony'.[59] There is every reason to think that Jenner did indeed publish it. A letter survives that clearly indicates the existence of a substantial manuscript, too long for 'quarto form', sent to an unscrupulous character called Dibdin. Jenner demanded complete secrecy in employing Dibdin to find a publisher.[60] Jenner scholars have known about this letter for decades, but have not been able to identify any publication of this type that could be attributed to Jenner. The prospect of finding the anonymously published pamphlet – evidence of Jenner's spirited engagement with the gutter – has whet the appetite of Jenner scholars for years, but nobody has worked out what, if anything, was published. This mystery can now be laid to rest.

The pamphlet *Letters to Dr Rowley* appeared in 1805, in octavo form, published by Symonds and printed by

Norris (also favoured by Jenner's allies). The author chose a pointed pseudonym for his sharp words: Aculeus. The evidence indicates that this is Jenner's anonymous pamphlet. It is published in the right year and in the right format. It is in 'letter' form, as Baron stated. The introduction, echoing Baron's diction, states that Rowley's work was 'totally unworthy a serious reply' and sets out 'to ridicule' him.[61] As per the letter to Dibdin, it goes out of its way explicitly to mention the 'Men of consequence who have figured on the Vaccine side', attaching honour to those names Rowley had threatened to besmirch.[62] It refers, both in the introduction and the appendix, to the work and reputation of Dr Thornton, who was Jenner's correspondent at the time concerning the anti-vaccinationist attacks. Thornton himself published his own pamphlet in the following year (Aculeus even notes that it is forthcoming) containing an extract of one of Jenner's letters that was remarkably close to the exasperation of Aculeus. Both bemoan the pointlessness of argument with an inoculator hypocrite:

> who plainly tells you he has made up his opinion, and believes it an act of gross *impiety* to inoculate for the *Cow-pock*, as interfering with the decrees of Heaven, while, at the same time, he himself is inoculating for the *Small-pox*, and boasts his partial success in this very interference, namely, the abating of mortality by a NEW METHOD! To argue with a person of this description, would be beating the air.[63]

In its introduction and appendix it is consistently Jennerian in tone when compared with his correspondence of this time. And finally, in accord with Baron's observation, it does indeed contain a 'great deal of wit and polished irony'.[64] More conclusive proof is unlikely to be forthcoming, but the circumstantial evidence is overwhelmingly persuasive.

Jenner's anonymous work was generally favourably received. It must have gratified him enormously to have finally been able to pour scorn on his critics, to tarnish them with 'proof of insupportable vanity and self-conceit'.[65] Jenner wrote to Thornton of Rowley that he 'could pardon this kind of logic in an *old woman*', and indeed, Aculeus invents an old woman character, who denounces vaccination to the author while in the act of purchasing a copy of Gillray's print. Jenner reduced all the anti-vaccine noise to an outcry against the threat to the lucrative business of variolation, combined with the petty jealousies of those who resented his acknowledgement in Parliament.[66]

Of far more moment than the 'anti-vacks', as Jenner called them, were supposed friends who were actually more threatening to Jenner's reputation.[67] Chief among these, and the man who brought the worst out in Jenner, was George Pearson. After the debacle that had witnessed the contamination of cowpox virus with actual smallpox, Jenner sought to distance himself from the source of potential danger to the success of vaccination. Pearson was rash and ambitious, and made costly mistakes. The insult that followed the injury was in Pearson's attempt to steal Jenner's glory by being the first to establish an institution for vaccination in London. Pearson suggested some token role for Jenner, who saw only a transparent attempt to remove him to the sidelines. He responded by mocking the supposed 'honour' Pearson offered and reminded him that if the 'vaccine inoculation, from unguarded conduct, should sink into disrepute (and you must admit, Sir, that in more than one instance has its reputation suffered) I alone must bear the odium.' Pearson's 'unhandsome' conduct had convinced Jenner that he could 'never more have any private concerns with him.'[68] Moreover, Jenner took action to disrupt the patronage that Pearson had attracted and to bring support on to his own side. Within a year of the publication of the *Inquiry*, the mutual slinging of mud had begun.

Jenner immediately set about planning his own institution, which came to nothing directly, but did prepare the way for the Royal Jennerian. The first action was to agitate directly against Pearson. Jenner had the advantage of personal audiences, so he was able to persuade Lord Egremont and the Duke of York to withdraw patronage from Pearson's scheme. The faintest whiff of dishonourable deeds on Pearson's part had the medical establishment flocking to Jenner's cause. If there were to be an institution at all, Jenner had determined that it would be by his own design.

Pearson was, perhaps understandably, disgruntled at having been disappointed in his ambitions. When it came to the discussion of Jenner's first Parliamentary award, Pearson went out of his way to testify that Jenner's petition should not be granted.[69] He combed the country for evidence that others had beaten Jenner to his discovery, that he was not worthy of public money, and did not deserve to be credited with priority. Although Pearson's evidence missed the point – nobody but Jenner had mastered human-to-human cowpox inoculations, and nobody else had broadcast the idea – it weighed heavily with Jenner that real enmity had quickly emerged. Parliament was not swayed by Pearson's testimony, but Jenner was ever afterwards guarded against those who might defame him. Pearson's proposed institution had stirred Jenner's increasingly proprietary attitude towards vaccination. While it is true that Jenner did not have pecuniary matters in mind when he published the *Inquiry*, it is fair to say that after the first Parliamentary grant Jenner became increasingly annoyed that he was not making his fortune from vaccination, even as others tried to snatch his glory and the income that came with it from under his nose.

In an audacious move, Pearson even tried to shift the blame for exporting the contaminated strain of cowpox to Europe on to Jenner, which infuriated him. Jenner worked his influence, writing to Alexander Marcet, the London-based but Swiss-born physician, to ask him to 'frustrate this malignant design' by writing to his European medical friends. Jenner felt that Pearson had 'endeavourd to fix an odium on me respecting the spurious Cow-Pox at Geneva'.[70]

He keenly felt the prick of false allies and fellow vaccinators, but the attacks of his anti-vaccinationist opponents generally passed him by. This can be witnessed in the internal strife at the Royal Jennerian, which Jenner observed with paranoid anxiety lest the practice of vaccination – and with it his name – be brought into disrepute. Here we see Jenner at his worst. He conducted the personnel operations of the Jennerian with a hatchet, when a scalpel was required. There was less of pre-eminence and more of prima donna about his presidency. In 1806 the various committees of the Royal Jennerian became embroiled in personal squabbling that completely distracted their focus from the job at hand. The resident vaccinator, John Walker, entered into a dispute with Jenner's friend Charles Murray, the secretary of the society. Murray accused Walker of breaking the seals of his mail. Walker, for his part, accused Murray of abusing the mail franking privileges of the society. Essentially, the honour of both was brought into question, but Walker was heavily censured. Later the same year, Walker was accused of bringing the Jennerian, and the practice of vaccination, into disrepute by introducing deviations from Jenner's own method, which was supposed to be a non-negotiable dogma of the society.

Jenner was present in London for some of the meetings, but for the most part he was informed of goings-on by letter and dictated policy by the same means. Jenner and his allies on the committee came to realise that Walker was the wrong man for the job, but the good name of the society and of Jenner himself were needlessly and publicly dragged through the mud in the affair to get rid of him. Jenner had a letter placed on the minutes in July 1806 detailing 'the grounds on which I have long founded my opinion that Dr Walker is incompetent to discharge the duties of the important office to which he has been appointed'. He considered Walker's published opinions on vaccination, which hardly anybody had noticed, to have 'disgraced the society'. 'What will the Publick think on comparing the instruction given by Dr Walker with those given by me, when they find them so different in many essential points[?]', Jenner asked. Jenner wished to be 'exonerated from any farther responsibility for his conduct' and threatened to resign as president of the Medical Council unless Walker was sacked. At the next meeting Jenner was present to ensure that a resolution was passed that Walker had 'very materially deviated' from Jenner's own designs. In a resolution, the committee thanked Jenner 'for the open minded, liberal and zealous manner in which he has exerted himself upon every occasion to support the best interests of this society'. Thus the cowering committee puffed up their champion. Walker's dismissal took place in the open court sessions of the society, in which Jenner and his allies ensured that Walker could not be saved, though he was not without support. This blunt-instrument style of management had turned colleagues into warring factions. Jenner confided to Marcet that he was suspicious of military manoeuvres, having sent spurious flags of truce from Walker 'back to the Enemys [*sic*] camp'.[71]

Walker left in disgrace but did not go quietly. He immediately formed a rival vaccination society, which he established in the same London square as the Royal Jennerian, using Jenner's name to attract patronage away from Jenner's own society. This was scurrilous behaviour and Jenner mobilised his forces to batter Walker's new institution. Every peer, MP, bishop and 'dignified clergy' was petitioned to send money and warned against the new institution. A circular letter was sent to all the subscribers of Walker's establishment warning them of his 'gross misconduct'.[72] Jenner had acquired the connections and the means to attempt to control the vaccination narrative and to shut down opponents. He never lost sight of the humanitarian cause, but it was always bound up with the protection of his good name.

Pearson, meanwhile, had resorted to new depths to defame Jenner and was even moving towards the camp of the anti-vaccinationists. In Jenner's eyes, Pearson had tried to make a career of attempting to 'ruin my reputation' one way or another. He was 'a very great Rogue; but so hardened that nothing can reform him'.[73] This brings us back to the formation of the National Vaccine Establishment, and why its foundation was, for Jenner, more galling than glorious. For nearly six months during 1808 Jenner stayed in London, which he loathed. It made him miserable company and he saw enemies everywhere. He felt isolated, and even close friends were suspected of a lack of fidelity. In an extraordinary series of letters to his close friend and ally, Thomas Pruen, Jenner revealed an increasing sense of unease, coupled with an unpleasant strain of self-piteous anxiety. The series begins with Jenner's foreboding about having to depart his pastoral repose, to 'go to a place ... I abhor beyond all others'. He feared the 'abominable Taunts' and forecast that his 'nerves will curl up like Fiddle strings' in front of a hot fire. To Jenner, the opportunity to personally guide the foundation of the National Vaccine Establishment was a 'sentence of Transportation'. The price of fame was punishment, squabbling and dislocation from family.[74]

In London in the spring of 1808, Jenner soon became miserably lonely, 'insulated from my friends – spending restless days & sleepless nights'. He understood the task at hand as one requiring a hero, but felt hopelessly inadequate. He was 'Look'd up to as one fit to erect a state Pillar, without any knowledge of such kind of Architecture'. He could see nothing but a 'situation ... wretched ... beyond anything I have before experience'd – from hurry & confusion'. His heart and spirit were 'broken, from the cruel privations' of London. In isolated vexation, he had a heightened awareness of the naysayers. In early July he chided Pruen for a lack of material support. He perceived his opponents 'by the most abominable falsities', endeavouring 'to ruin my private character'. So much he could bear, 'but when I find that no friend has step'd forth even to hold an Umbrella over my head it makes me feel miserable'.[75]

A new issue of the *Medical Observer* 'cramm'd with antivaccine Rubbish' came to his attention in September.

The old foe Birch included a print of 'four Heads *diseas'd by Vaccination*'. He might, Jenner thought, 'have added his own & made a fifth'. Jenner was afraid, but for the moment in control of his fear: 'I *know* from good information that my person is not in safety here, yet I do not feel the least dread of assassination.' He was locked in the stocks, unable to avoid the abuse and waiting for the bureaucratic glacier to move to a favourable position: 'How little did I imagine that the galling fetters which the Public have forged for me would still have remained so firmly lock'd.' The arrangements for the National Vaccine Establishment dragged on slowly; by late October Jenner thought it 'a shocking piece of business' that he was still in town; by late November he could scarcely credit it. He spiralled into a doleful whine, bemoaning his lot. While his '*happy* discovery' had excited 'sensations of the most pleasurable kind', these had been counterbalanced by sensations of the opposite order.[76] He returned home to Berkeley with nothing fixed.

Matters took a turn for the worse. As the establishment took shape, Jenner quickly felt the sting of being sidelined and slighted: 'The Board appointed me Director of course, but they have contriv'd to let me know that I am the Director directed.' Jenner had put forward eight names to fill the principal vaccinating stations, but all except two were rejected. This was despite earlier assurances that his judgement was to be final in this regard.[77] To make matters worse, 'indeed is it not insulting?' Jenner asked, 'one of them who is appointed the Vaccine Chief … is really taken from Pearsons [*sic*] Institution, to which he was Surgeon.' This was the 'very man who linkd himself with Pearson to form his Institution, & the very man who made a base attempt to upset me in the Committee of the House of Commons'.[78] The man in question, Joseph Carpue, was perfectly respectable, but tainted in Jenner's eyes. The spectre of Pearson again loomed over Jenner's reputation, and he could not stomach it. Even more bewildering, the appointment was at the expense of John Ring, who had championed Jenner since the *Inquiry* and who was a doyen of Jenner's method.[79] Unfortunately, Ring had also been the chief rabble-rouser, doing battle in the gutter with the anti-vaccinationists. This partisan choice by Jenner had proven particularly injudicious. The medical establishment, represented by the Royal College of Surgeons and the Royal College of Physicians, both of which had significant influence in the formation of the new institution, was exerting its authority.

What to do? Resign immediately, or wait a while and then resign? His plaintive cry for help, in the context of months of self-indulgent complaint, inevitably fell on deaf ears. Jenner, paranoid, spelled out his dilemma:

By submission, what am I but an underling in an Institution in which Pearson will, thro his agents virtually take the lead; and to resist & thereby gain my point, will throw me upon a bed of Vipers; for not only those who by a struggle on my part may be dismiss'd, but their numerous adherents, will be for ever wounding me with their Fangs. I may most piteously exclaim, what shall I do?[80]

Jenner had allowed vaccination to slip to second place in his priorities behind the cause of public esteem for Edward Jenner, and Pruen rebuffed him curtly: 'I am sorry for your situation, but can afford you no kind of assistance.' Not only had vaccination proved to be a source of 'embarassment [sic] & vexation' for Jenner, instead of comfort, now even his friends could not be relied upon to lend succour. Jenner went ahead and resigned from the new establishment, causing chaos in its early organisation. Jenner referred to Pruen's conduct as a 'dead Cut', becoming petulant. He scolded his friend and further bemoaned his luck:

What if a Man had met with an old Friend who had tumbled into a Cellar or any other kind of pit & had broke his bones & had pass'd by heedless of his moanings, saying I am sorry for you but cannot stay to help you out, because I have a pressing engagement, that I must attend to in another quarter? Would this have been balsam to his Wounds or a Caustic? Sufficient – I am to be torn limb from limb it seems by Government & the College of Phys: but I hope my Executors will collect my scatterd remains and give me Christian burial. Hostilities are about to commence, & the odds against me would be fearful if my Heart was not well shielded – but I have nothing to reproach myself with, tho much to be vext at. I shall not trouble you by going into particulars, but only say, that the new Institution is disgraceful to the Nation & degrading to me.[81]

It was actually neither of these things, as Jenner later came to realise. By June of 1809, he acknowledged that the new establishment was flourishing, but still thought its 'framers treat me with dishonour'. Some years later he congratulated Charles Murray on 'the most satisfactory and impressive' report of the establishment's activities, which had gone further than 'any Society since the introduction of Vaccination'. Jenner wanted to pat the director on the back and 'call him a good Fellow', but doubted the compliment would be returned.[82] He rediscovered his humility late in the day, when the institution of vaccination was better established and his service to humanity was, if not recognised by the populace, at least properly acknowledged by the medical community. He continued to feel the ingratitude of his own country, compared with the fame he had found abroad, and at the end of his life he still found it necessary to draw up and circulate a memorandum on the utility, and more importantly the method, of vaccination.[83] But by then the worst had passed. At the time of the foundation of the National Vaccine Establishment and the demise of the Royal Jennerian, Jenner's ego, heightened sense of honour and constant looking over his shoulder had made him unpopular in all quarters. He was about to be plagued by greater and more personal concerns.

6

Tragedy

My Spirits are for the most part miserably low, &
I must expect they will remain so, till the few verses
that remain of the Chapter are ended.

Edward Jenner, 1816[84]

Jenner contemplated with equanimity the lives that vaccination had saved. He was acutely aware of the impact of his work but seemed only nominally proud. He grounded himself in simple pleasures and a parsimonious domestic life. At the same time, he despised those who continued with inoculation or otherwise denied the power of the cowpox at least as much for the damage this did to his reputation as for the human cost of ignorance. Although Jenner was himself inoculated as a child, his own life might be thought of as relatively untouched by smallpox. Certainly he encountered it frequently enough, and until he began vaccinating in the 1790s he was actively inoculating his patients with smallpox, as was the norm. But from 1796 onwards, Jenner's dealings with smallpox were, on the whole, focused on prevention; the people he saw were healthy and stayed that way. He gladly received news of vaccination from around the world and took reports of smallpox outbreaks as an impetus for his own vaccination campaign. It is impossible to calculate the number of lives he saved, but what was this to Jenner when faced with suffering close to home, with diseases he did not understand and could not prevent, and with the deaths of those he held dearest?

It is easy to look back on Jenner's life and assume that his assault on smallpox was what he intended for his life's work. However, as the eclectic experimentation of his early professional years indicates, Jenner was a generalist, a tinkerer and insatiably curious. The success of vaccination and the difficulties he had to face as a result meant he no longer had the time to give a free rein to his curiosity; he often yearned for those earlier years when he had been able to indulge in seemingly inconsequential pursuits. When Jenner set out to discover something, he did not think through what might transpire if he were successful. Vaccination changed his life, almost against his will. However, if he had been able to choose the field of his success, perhaps it would not have been vaccination, but to understand the causes of tuberculosis and to develop a cure.

Early in his career, when he was killing cuckoos, losing thermometers inside hedgehogs and dissecting dogs, Jenner was also actively engaged in developing a theory of the causes of tuberculosis (this remained unknown in his lifetime; the bacillus responsible was only identified by Robert Koch in 1882). We might assume that such knowledge comes about procedurally, by following clear methods and with clear goals in mind. Yet controlled experiments are a distinctly modern affair; scientific discoveries have often been serendipitous, accidental and stumbled upon while looking for something entirely different. Jenner's work on vaccination is often hailed as one of the first, and therefore one of the exemplars, of controlled experimentation, with systematic verification built into the study. Nevertheless, Jenner did not actually know how vaccination worked – an understanding of the immune system that could explain the effect of cowpox would have to wait for the twentieth century – and his controlled methods were not applied to other areas of study. When looking at his efforts to find the cause of tuberculosis, the only similarity to his vaccination experiments is the conviction that he was absolutely right in his assertions. His research was by trial and error; his reasoning inductive.

Jenner was convinced that tuberculosis was caused by 'hydatids': parasitic larvae that caused pus-filled cysts. Jenner thought that the cysts he found in the lungs and other organs of various animals were themselves wormlike parasites. Indeed, cystic echinococcosis, or hydatid disease, is caused by tapeworms. Since the tubercles in the lungs looked like cysts, Jenner worked on the assumption that these too were related to worms. His assumption put tuberculosis in the same class of disorder as tumours of all kinds. According to Baron, Jenner 'laboured with unceasing perseverance to throw light upon the subject, earnestly hoping that accurate knowledge on the origin and progress of this class of diseases would lead to more successful means of treating them'.[85] The idealism and altruistic humanity characterised by Baron is typical enough, but it is likely that Jenner had other motivations. As Baron noted, Catharine Jenner was not in the best of health, even before her marriage, and it became commonly known in Jenner's circle by as early as 1804 that she was 'seized with spitting of blood'.[86] Even if the onset of tuberculosis only became apparent to Jenner at this time, it would undoubtedly have concentrated his efforts, although he was already working on worms by 1790. The disease that hung threateningly over the Jenner household was not smallpox, but TB.

In 1790 Jenner had presented to his peers at the Gloucestershire Medical Society a paper on the subject of hydatids in the kidneys and the use of the essential oil of turpentine to remove them.[87] For once, Hunter wasn't supportive of this notion, though Baron took up the work and tried to make something out of it.[88] Jenner wrote in his own notes, undated but probably in the mid-1790s, that he had 'long ago conceived that the true tuberculous consumption originated in hydatids getting into the lungs & there forming tubercles'. Once again, he was led into morbid anatomy and dissection, but the fauna was getting bigger. He sliced into what he identified as tubercles in the lungs of a cow and examined the watery fluid that emerged, finding in it 'about twenty hydatids'. He wondered if the cyst itself was a hydatid, reproducing German research that had already been carried out, but that Jenner had almost certainly not seen. Local circumstances afforded him every opportunity to study this phenomenon, since his butcher slaughtered a couple of fat oxen every other day. For weeks on end, Jenner cut into the lungs of these animals, finding hydatids 'constantly'. The cysts, he tells us, varied in size, from that of a pea to that of a cricket ball, spurting out their contents when punctured. This fluid Jenner boiled to see if it coagulated (it did not) and tasted it (saltish)! He rushed to conclusions: 'may we not infer that encysted tumours in general are hydatids[?]'[89]

Jenner soon branched out, examining the lungs of hogs, sheep and finally humans. From where he acquired his tuberculous lungs is unknown, but by now he was firmly convinced that he was dealing with a common cause across the species barrier. The 'hydatid' he found in the lungs was full of 'a cheesy substance of a darkish colour' that reminded him of the hydatids of sheep. Was TB caused by 'our familiarity with an animal that nature intended to keep separate from man'?[90] The connection to his original thinking on cowpox was obvious. Maybe all human diseases could be so classified. He wrote his conclusions to his brother Henry, copying the letter for his own records; it expresses Jenner's energy and optimism that he had made a world-changing breakthrough:

> That species of consumption which arises from tubercles in the lungs is by far the most common & the most fatal to the human constitution. The appearance of tubercles in the lungs has been noticed from the ancient ages, but the cause in which they originate has not (as far as I know) been known or even guess'd at till now. From comparative dissections, that is, from comparing the diseas'd lungs of different quadrupeds with human lungs their origin has been clearly disclosed & it appears

to be owing to hydatids. The hydatid is a kind of insect (whose character I shall not now attempt to describe to you) that is capable of attaching itself to any part of the body, & producing diseased action in the surrounding parts. The diseas'd appearances, arising from this diseas'd action, vary according to the nature of the part to which the hydatid is attach'd. In the lungs this diseasd appearance has been call'd a tubercle. It exists after its exciting causes (the hydatid) has ceas'd to exist. It is commonly a kind of cyst* containing different substances. Some contain pus; in others there is gritty matter. In some of these cavities there is often a compact substance nearly of the consistence of congealed honey & now & then I find small hydatids floating in a limpid fluid within the same kind of cyst. The above is an imperfect sketch, but I much hope you will see in it my idea of the cause of the horrid malady pulmonary consumption.

The discovery, I trust, will introduce what has long been wanted – a new & better mode of treating the complaint – But still I despair of finding a remedy where it is far advanced, for nature has no process whereby she can regenerate portions of the lungs where destroyd by disease. Yet I by no means despair of discovering a preventive in what may be descried a consumptive constitution, or even a cure in the early stages.

*the cyst was originally an hydatid [91]

We know now that Jenner was wrong. He found a sympathetic ear in the Grand Duchess of Oldenburg, sister of Alexander I of Russia, whom he met in 1811.[92] Much as this flushed his pride, among his peers he found little encouragement. Some time around 1815 he wrote to Astley Cooper, the noted surgeon and anatomist, to remind him of his work on hydatids and tuberculosis. Jenner remembered that when he had first introduced Cooper to the subject Cooper had thought him 'whimsical', having 'dismissed the subject with a good humourd smile'. The next person Jenner told – possibly Sir Everard Home – 'vociferated so loud, & so hardly that he almost choak'd me by sending my words down my throat again'.[93] By this time Jenner had lived with his understanding of tuberculosis for at least twenty-five years. For the smallpox hero, such ridicule must have been difficult to bear.

The intellectual and reputational burden of being wrong, however, was nothing compared to the personal cost. In 1806 Jenner employed a young man called John Worgan to tutor his son Edward. By 1809 Worgan was dead of tuberculosis. The disease was definitively in the Jenner household, and it would continue to wreak havoc. Edward was the next to fall ill, and Jenner had to endure his first-born's illness from a distance, at least at the beginning. Stuck in hateful London at the end of 1808, dealing with the interminable affairs surrounding the foundation of the National Vaccine Establishment, Jenner looked for comfort in news from home and found little. 'Poor Edward is again going through one of his dreadful

Fevers', he told his friend Pruen. He set off home with 'a heavy Heart' and hoped only to 'shut myself in my Cottage, & quit it no more. The world is not worth a farthing.' Once home he found Edward convalescent and he rejoiced, but the relief was temporary and disturbed by Edward's 'little cough' and 'too quick a pulse'.[94]

Sometime in the middle of 1809, 'Poor Edward's complaint which remained so long enveloped in obscurity' finally revealed itself 'in a most alarming shape'. Haemorrhaging from the lungs, the weak young man was discharging profuse amounts of blood every two or three days. Jenner tried to be phlegmatic, at least in his letters, for while 'Death is a terrible visitor in whatever shape he approaches us', he could not argue against 'God's will'. Yet the sound of Edward's 'hollow cough' plunged Jenner into a miserable depression.[95] In October he told his friend Dr Morgan of his slump into melancholy and despair: 'My poor Boy still exists, but is wasting inch by inch. The ray of Hope is denied only to a medical Man when he sees his Child dying of pulmonary Consumption; all other Mortals enjoy its flattering light.' In early 1810, Edward died, his father noting that he had taken with him 'much of my earthly comfort'. Again Jenner looked to the omnipresent God who had willed this event, but he was devastated. He had had 'no conception till it happened that the gash would have been so deep', he told his friend Hicks, further wondering to John Ring why the mind is not reconciled to an inevitable event 'when it has made such gradual approaches'. Jenner lamented, 'the edge of sensibility is not thus to be blunted'.[96] Again and again the sigh, God's will be done, God's will be done.

In 1815 Catharine went the same way. Her health throughout her life had been poor, but a sudden decline took her from Jenner in September; sources generally agree that tuberculosis was the underlying cause. She had probably had it for years, but the end was still a 'severe shock' to Jenner. She had been confined to her room for much of her final summer with Jenner in Cheltenham, but a fateful walk about the streets exposed her to a chill, and bronchitis set in on top of her 'usual pulmonic symptoms'.[97] Stunned into wretchedness, Jenner retreated immediately from Cheltenham, setting himself up at home in Berkeley for good. He never really went anywhere again.

From his seclusion he wrote of the need for company, craving the sympathy of others as the only tonic for his private suffering. Alone, surrounded by the emotive objects of his domestic content, he was continually reminded of his 'irreparable loss', yet unable to quit his own walls. He begged Baron to come and exercise his pity. He told another friend, Dr Burder, that there was a 'secret Charm in sympathy', 'soothing … the wounded spirit'. When friends exhibited a 'feeling Heart' it consoled his 'sensations of the most painful kind', the privations that 'cut deep'. But all of this was so much rhetoric, a discourse of sensibility that he strove to make true. The reality was bleak. Part of Edward Jenner had ceased to be, and the part that remained was 'in a sad sad state of decomposition'. True to the eighteenth-century medical philosophy that he had carried with him throughout his life, Jenner believed that the 'mind & body act reciprocally on each other' and thought that the transformations in each had made him a different creature. To Pruen, his closest correspondent, he entertained scant hope of a revival: 'My Spirits are for the most part miserably low, & I must expect they will remain so, till the few verses that remain of the Chapter are ended.'[98]

By and large, that was how the chapter played out. Jenner was still animated by the cause of vaccination, but the abstract suffering of populations unknown to him, and even his own reputation, became less important than his own pain, mental and physical, and his fears for his surviving family. The saviour of millions looked about him and saw little evidence that the predation of disease was any less of a threat for all his efforts. Even Phipps, the boy who had received the famous first vaccination, eventually succumbed, as a pauper adult, to tuberculosis.[99] Jenner worried about the health of his second son, Robert, then at Oxford. The 'mists & clouds' enveloped him in a melancholy state and he complained of solitude, which 'sinks one into the Earth'.[100] He suffered various illnesses that kept him low for months on end, and probably had his first stroke in the summer of 1820.[101] Thereafter he developed an acute auditory hyperaesthesia, which perhaps betokened the onset of more serious neurological conditions. Contemporary medicine struggles to understand such phenomena, and in Jenner's time this condition was an impenetrable mystery.

This illness, which Jenner assumed (aptly) to be a 'mechanical' fault somewhere in the brain, turned what was left of his domestic contentment into a form of hell. He complained to Baron that he could not bear the 'sharp sounds elicited by the sudden contact' of knives and forks on plates and glasses. These noises were violent shocks to his system. He was unfazed by church bells or thunder, but the 'clatter of a dinner Table is worst of all'. He begged Marcet to think of a remedy, knowing not what to do with himself: 'In a Female I should call it Hysterical – but in myself I know not what to call it, but by the old sweeping term nervous. Will you allow me to call it electrical?' And to Parry he wished for the days of the 'wooden Spoon & Trencher', that would 'smooth the tide of life'. Succour was not forthcoming. On the morning of 25 January 1823, Jenner suffered a massive stroke. Baron found him, having been placed in bed, apoplectic and half paralysed. At about 3 a.m. the next day, Jenner breathed his last.[102]

7

Legacy

Yours is the comfortable reflection that mankind can
never forget that you have lived.

Thomas Jefferson, 1806[103]

Jenner did not single-handedly ensure a global protection against smallpox, but his work and his name fostered revolutionary changes that would bolster armies and empires, and ensure the survival of distant colonies and ravaged urban centres. The rapid eradication of smallpox among those who availed themselves of vaccination changed the concept of beauty, diminishing the ubiquity of facial scarring that had been an inevitable part of life. It also changed the emotional lives of children and parents, who rested easy in the knowledge that the fearful monster smallpox was no longer biding its time, waiting to pluck the innocent.

It was not a straight road to success, and the journey was not complete by the time of Jenner's death. He did not understand why or how vaccination worked, and he did not know that a single vaccination was not sufficient to protect for life. On both these points, a dogmatic and doctrinaire stubbornness hindered his vision, but these qualities were probably necessary to shore up the practice against his bitter enemies, who stoked the fires of fear among the population. Nevertheless, vaccination in 1823 was on the wane. Smallpox continued to ravage, despite the profound evidence of vaccination's utility. The Jenner we have come to know – celebrated, heroic, giant – had a questionable reputation for decades after his death. His friends, meanwhile, tried to reify and immortalise his beneficence. Jenner was to be set in stone, cast in bronze, fired in terracotta. To make a hero out of a contested reputation in Regency and early Victorian Britain, there was no better way than to commission a statue.

Numerous statues of Jenner remain around the world, but the two most famous stand in Gloucester Cathedral and in Kensington Gardens. The one in Gloucester owes its existence to the activism of Baron – there was no finer hero-worshipper than he – and Jenner's Masonic lodge, but paid for by subscriptions, which were apparently slow in coming. It is, considering Jenner's preference for the locale, a fitting tribute, but it is somewhat out of the way. The other statue was the idea of a career-minded sculptor by the name of Calder Marshall who sought out subscribers and found support, with some difficulty, in the USA and Russia, and in the deep pockets of Prince Albert. Jenner was put in pride of place in Trafalgar Square in 1858. He lasted all of four years before being moved to Kensington Gardens, banished as too controversial a figure, despite the protestations of the medical community.[104] Why was he banished?

There had been rumblings of annoyance among radicals from the start. Thomas Duncombe thought Jenner out of place 'among statues of our naval and military heroes', but his objection had more to do with Jenner being the 'promulgator of cow-pock nonsense'.[105] In that statement, Duncombe captured the popular mood in an era in which vaccination had been made compulsory by law. The almost unanimous support of the medical community for Jenner's innovation had been brought to bear, and the State was making unprecedented inroads into the private lives of its citizens. The original humanitarian spark that Jenner had fanned into a worldwide flame of benevolence was suddenly perceived by many as the hellfire of invidious government, burning precious liberties and risking the lives of children against the wishes of their parents. How had it come to such a dramatic polarisation of opinion, and why did Jenner the villain seem to be in the ascendency?

Two significant Acts of Parliament were chiefly responsible for tarnishing Jenner's reputation. The first, in 1840, was prompted by a major epidemic.[106] It made smallpox inoculation (variolation) illegal and made vaccination freely available for anyone who wanted it. Jenner had campaigned for the outlawing of inoculation during his lifetime, but without success; the livelihoods of too many medical celebrities depended on their capacity to give people a light dose of the smallpox for a fee. The public health argument – that smallpox by inoculation was just as contagious as smallpox acquired in the natural way – eventually won out in the face of widespread suffering. The State intervened to ensure the protection of the population at large, over the claims of individuals. Since vaccination provided a safe alternative to inoculation, it made no sense to continue to allow the medical profession to put the health of the people at risk.

The second significant piece of legislation came in 1853. The Vaccination Act made vaccination compulsory for all newborn babies in the land.[107] This Act is a landmark piece of legislation for a number of reasons. It was the first assertion of State power in relation to health provision on a universal basis. Some mark it as the opening gambit on the way to socialised medicine and the National Health Service.[108] More sinister, perhaps, than universal provision was universal compulsion. In the two decades that followed the 1853 Vaccination Act, the law would be increasingly tightened in order to punish parents who allowed their children to remain unvaccinated. Free choice or conscientious objection were strictly prohibited. Parents who broke the law were prosecuted, fined and commanded to comply. If they refused they were prosecuted again. In lieu of fines that could not be paid, some households had their goods distrained. Other parents were sent to prison. When the law was at its harshest, the sentence came with hard labour. Fears of vaccination, combined with claims about its potential ill effects – syphilis, erysipelas, etc. – were summarily dismissed by magistrates who followed the letter of the law.

A more cynical problem concerned the machinery of vaccination practices. Responsibility for delivering vaccination in England was put in the hands of the Poor Law Guardians, which had the unfortunate (from the point of view of the middle classes and beyond) effect of associating vaccination with the workhouse. What respectable mother would take her child to be contaminated with matter drawn from the arm of a ne'er-do-well? Cowpox was one thing, but what about all the other diseases that riddled the poor? Social stratification, the class system, relied on bodies being kept apart. The State's insistence on bringing bodies together seemed, to those for whom the workhouse was a symbol of shame, to risk the fabric of civilisation.[109]

An extensive Parliamentary commission of inquiry was undertaken towards the end of the nineteenth century to try to establish the efficacy of vaccination once and for all. This did ultimately result in some softening of the clause relating to compulsion, but the conclusion of the commission was firmly in favour of Jenner's discovery. Caveats were included. The need for revaccination was now commonly acknowledged. Vaccination in infancy worked, but only for a few years, after which it was necessary to top up the immune system. More importantly, perhaps, was the discursive wrangling over statistics that seemed at once to prove and disprove the prophylactic power of vaccination. Some well-known figures, most notably the co-discoverer of evolution by natural selection, Alfred Russel Wallace, came out as fierce anti-vaccinationists. Others, like Charles Darwin, thought the anti-vaccinationists 'bigots'.[110] Medical debate was not being driven by an intricate working knowledge, but by results, which were themselves full of uncertainty. Wallace had provocatively asserted that Jenner had lived in 'a pre-scientific age', but the acrimony over vaccination seemed to bring the scientific credo of Wallace's own age into question.[111] While the compilers of statistics in favour of the practice had the last word, and a more impressive array of numbers than could be produced by the anti-vaccinationists, what was eminently clear was that nobody precisely understood how vaccination worked. While vaccination as a practice ultimately prevailed, and remained compulsory in England throughout the last half of the nineteenth century, the public was not inclined to celebrate its discoverer. To have Jenner in pride of place in Trafalgar Square might have risked a riot.

This is no exaggeration. Anti-vaccination riots consumed whole towns (Leicester in 1885 was a prime example) and some local Guardians began to defy the law. Better knowledge of how contagion worked led to alternative proposals to isolate smallpox cases and thereby prevent major outbreaks without resorting to vaccination. Less crowded urban spaces with improved sanitation seemed to promise a healthier future, with no need of Jenner's vaccine. The future of medicine, from a popular point of view, lay in clean air and clean streets, not in the tainting of human blood with animal viruses.

Such was the popular mood. Fortunately for Jenner's legacy, and for humanity at large, it was not shared by medical scientists. Jenner was the inspiration for continued research on the immune systems of humans and animals. A central thesis – that cowpox was a weakened form of smallpox, which provided immunity without serious infection – was developed into a research agenda that would see Louis Pasteur engineer 'vaccines' for cholera, anthrax and rabies. This label – 'vaccine' – that we now apply to all prophylactic inoculations, whether for mumps, measles, influenza or, most recently, Ebola, stems from Pasteur wishing to honour Jenner's work. The medical legacy of Jenner's discovery, and his equally important forays into the administration of public health, is now most clearly evident in national and international efforts to prevent all manner of diseases. Jenner is justly known as the father of immunology, a science which has had a profound and positive impact on human and animal health and, as a result, significantly reduced the amount of money needed to cope with the effects of disease. Medicine, with Jenner, shifted its gaze from cure to prevention.

Smallpox is, essentially, extinct. It exists in secure locations in the USA and Russia: hidden vials of fear that keep its threat present amid 'continued uncertainty over its ownership'. The World Health Organization (WHO) spearheaded the campaign to put an end to the disease, with great success, but it retains tens of millions of doses of vaccine, just in case.[112] Enduring fears of a smallpox weapon or the re-emergence of the disease via other nefarious means should not overshadow the scale of the achievement in eliminating smallpox. The WHO's eradication campaign began in 1958 and intensified in 1966. At this time the disease was still a major problem in certain parts of the world, especially in what we now call the 'developing world'. The WHO co-ordinated the delivery of vaccines, observation, isolation, notification and diagnosis across the world, documenting the last case of smallpox in each country. The last ever case of smallpox was in Somalia. With the patient's recovery, 'smallpox zero' was declared on 26 October 1979.[113] Smallpox remains one of only two diseases that have been completely eliminated as a direct result of medical research and public health activism (the other being rinderpest in 2011). Edward Jenner is the father of the greatest single medical achievement in the history of humanity. Though disconnected from the final victory over smallpox by more than a century and a half, it is fair to point out that from the very beginning Jenner had the complete annihilation of smallpox as his aim.[114] It was a grand, noble vision that has since been matched by a grand, noble effort.

Jenner seems now to be assured of giant status. In 2002, he was voted the seventy-eighth greatest Briton of all time in a popular BBC poll. Such things are not important in their own right, but it is extraordinary that, in a list heavily skewed toward the recent past and to celebrity, this eighteenth-century rural doctor found his place. The forecast of Thomas Jefferson, who said of Jenner in 1806, 'Yours is the comfortable reflection that mankind can never forget that you have lived,' was accurate.[115] More recently, Gareth Williams attempted to reinvigorate interest in putting Jenner's Kensington Gardens statue back in Trafalgar Square.[116] The campaign failed, but perhaps this is of little consequence; there is no longer the same popular taste for memorialising heroes in bronze. Jenner's achievements and his legacy are better marked by a profound absence. Look around at the faces of people, at their eyes, at the smooth skin of children. The once ubiquitous bodily scarring of smallpox is unknown to us. There can be no better monument to Jenner than humanity itself.

Timeline

1749	17 May: Born, eighth of nine children. Father Stephen was vicar of Berkeley
c. 1763	Apprenticed for seven years to Daniel Ludlow, surgeon
1770	Moves to London, completes medical training at St George's under John Hunter
1772	Becomes local surgeon/physician at Berkeley
1788	Elected Fellow of the Royal Society for his work on the life of the cuckoo Marries Catharine Kingscote
1789	First son, Edward, born
1792	Made MD, University of St Andrews
1796	Performs first human-to-human inoculation of cowpox on 8-year-old James Phipps, later inoculating him (without infecting him) with smallpox
1798	Publishes *An Inquiry into the Causes and Effects of the Variolæ Vaccinæ*
1799	Published *Further Observations on the Variolæ Vaccinæ, or Cow-Pox*

1800	Publishes *A Continuation of Facts and Observations relative to the Variolæ Vaccinæ*
1802	Parliamentary grant awarded, £10,000
1803	Jennerian Society founded
1807	Parliamentary grant awarded, £20,000
1808	National Vaccine Establishment founded. Jenner soon resigns to defend his honour
1810	Loses his eldest son to tuberculosis
1815	Sudden death of his wife, also of tuberculosis
1821	Appointed physician-extraordinary to George IV
1823	Submits 'Observations on the Migration of Birds' to the Royal Society
1823	26 January: Dies of a stroke
1840	Smallpox inoculation banned by Act of Parliament
1853	Vaccination made compulsory by law in England and Wales
1889–96	Royal Commission on Vaccination, takes testimony from around the world. Results in broad vindication of the practice, but compulsion is ultimately relaxed
1966	World Health Organization (WHO) launches major campaign to eradicate smallpox
1979	WHO declares smallpox 'dead'

Abbreviations

RCS   Royal College of Surgeons of England
RCP   Royal College of Physicians of England
RSM   Royal Society of Medicine, London
BL   British Library, London
WL   Wellcome Library, London

Notes

1   Baron, J., *The Life of Edward Jenner*, 2 volumes (Henry Colburn, 1838), vol. 2, p. 315.

2   Ibid., vol. 2, p. 315.

3   Fisher, R.B., *Edward Jenner: A Biography* (Andre Deutsch, 1991).

4   Fosbroke, T.D., *Berkeley Manuscripts* (John Nichols, 1821), p. 222; Baron, *Life*, vol. 1, p. 3.

5   Hunter to Jenner, 2 August [1775], RCS HUN: J 49.G.18 Hunter to Jenner, Letters 1773–93.

6   Jenner, E., 'Observations on the Natural History of the Cuckoo', *Philosophical Transactions of the Royal Society of London*, 78 (1788), pp. 219–37.

7   Hunter to Jenner, n.d. [1777], RCS HUN: J 49.G.18 Hunter to Jenner, Letters 1773–93.

8   Hunter to Jenner, 2 August [1775], RCS HUN: J 49.G.18 Hunter to Jenner, Letters 1773–93.

9   Jenner, 'Observations', p. 223.

10 Hunter to Jenner, [12 April 1777 and 16 April 1777], RCS HUN: J 49.G.18 Hunter to Jenner, Letters 1773–93; Jenner to G. Cumberland, 8 February 1819, BL Add MS 36507 f. 38.

11 Hunter to Jenner [July 1778], RCS HUN: J 49.G.18
    Hunter to Jenner, Letters 1773–93.

12 Hunter to Jenner, 25 September 1778, RCS HUN:
    J 49.G.18 Hunter to Jenner, Letters 1773–93.

13 Baron, *Life*, vol. 1, p. 52.

14 Jenner, 'Observations', p. 232.

15 Ibid., p. 228.

16 Baron, *Life*, vol. 1, pp. 148–9.

17 For example, WL MS 3018 diary with patient notes
    [for 1794].

18 Jenner, E., 'Some Observations on the Migration
    of Birds', *Philosophical Transactions of the Royal
    Society of London*, vol. 114 (1824), pp. 11–44. For
    experiments on dogs and emetic tartar see RCP
    MS372, Edward Jenner Diary; RCS HUN:J 49.G.18
    Hunter to Jenner, Letters 1773–93.

19 Baron, *Life*, vol. 1, p. 87.

20 Hunter to Jenner, 31 Mar 1789, RCS HUN: J 49.G.18
    Hunter to Jenner, Letters 1773–93.

21 RCP MS736, Regulations and Transactions of the
    Glocestershire [*sic*] Medical Society Instituted May
    1788; see minute of 30 July 1788 and Jenner's *Angina
    pectoris* MS on f. 11.

22 Parry, C., *An Inquiry into the Symptoms and Causes
    of the Syncope Anginosa, Commonly Called Angina
    Pectoris* (Cruttwell, 1799), pp. 3–6, 108–10. Dudley
    Hart, F., 'William Heberden, Edward Jenner, John
    Hunter and Angina Pectoris', *Journal of Medical
    Biography*, 3 (1995), pp. 56–8.

23   Jenner to Phillips, 16 January 1807, RCP MS 735, f. 22.

24   Li, Y., Carroll, D.S., Gardner S.N. et al., 'On the Origin of Smallpox: Correlating Variola Phylogenics with Historical Smallpox Records', *Proceedings of the National Academy of Sciences of the United States of America*, 104 (2007), pp. 15787–92; Hughes, A.L., Irausquin, S. & Friedman, R., 'The Evolutionary Biology of Poxviruses', *Infection, Genetics and Evolution*, 10 (2010), pp. 50–9; Riedel, S., 'Edward Jenner and the History of Smallpox and Vaccination', *Baylor University Medical Center Proceedings*, 18 (2005), pp. 21–5, p. 21.

25   Grundy, I., *Lady Mary Wortley Montagu: Comet of the Enlightenment* (Oxford University Press, 1999).

26   Riedel, 'Edward Jenner', p. 22; Williams, G., *Angel of Death: The Story of Small Pox* (Palgrave Macmillan, 2010), pp. 28–148.

27   Fosbroke, *Berkeley Manuscripts*, pp. 221–2.

28   Jenner to Gardner, 19 July 1796, RCS Box MS0016 4 & 6, Edward Jenner [miscellaneous].

29   Baron, *Life*, vol. 1, p. 122.

30   Ibid., vol. 1, p. 48; Jenner, G.C., *The Evidence at Large, as Laid Before the Committee of the House of Commons, Respecting Dr. Jenner's Discovery of Vaccine Inoculation* (J. Murray, 1805), p. 11; RCP MS736, Regulations and Transactions of the Glocestershire [*sic*] Medical Society Instituted May 1788, 20 June 1790, f. 12.

31   Baron, *Life*, vol. 1, p. 130–1.

32   RCS MS0016/1, *An Inquiry into the Natural History of a Disease known in Glostershire by the name of the Cow-pox* (Jenner's original MS).

33   Jenner to Gardner, 19 July 1796, RCS Box MS0016 4 & 6, Edward Jenner [miscellaneous].

34   Letter to the editors, *London Medical and Physical Journal*, 3 (1800), p. 102.

35   Jenner, E., *An Inquiry into the Causes and Effects of the Variolæ Vaccinæ, a Disease Discovered in Some of the Western Counties of England … Known by the Name of the Cow Pox* (London, 1798), p. 1.

36   Moseley, B., *A Treatise on Sugar, with Miscellaneous Medical Observations* (2nd edn, John Nichols, 1800), p. 183.

37   Jenner to Mrs Black [1807] WL MS 5226/5.

38   Baron, *Life*, vol. 2, pp. 449–57; Officer, L.H. & Williamson, S.H., 'Five Ways to Compute the Relative Value of a UK Pound Amount, 1270 to Present', MeasuringWorth, 2014, www.measuringworth. com/ukcompare; Fosbroke, *Berkeley Manuscripts*, pp. 237–8.

39   Baron, *Life*, vol. 2, pp. 101–5. See also W.R. LeFanu, *A Bio-Bibliography of Edward Jenner* (Harvey & Blythe, 1951), pp. 103–6.

40   Jenner to Hugh Scott, 14 September 1799, RCS Box MS0016 4 & 6, Edward Jenner [miscellaneous].

41   See, for example, Jenner to Lady Louisa Brome, 10 October 1801 and 7 December 1803, RCS Box

MS0016 4 & 6, Edward Jenner [miscellaneous];
Jenner to — of Leipzig, 5 July 1804, BL Add MS
39672: 1446-1864 f. 98; Baron, *Life*, vol. 2, p. 80.

42 Ibid., vol. 3, pp. 77–87; Jenner to Phillips, 16 January
1807, RCP MS 735, f. 22.

43 Baron, *Life*, vol. 1, pp. 393, 583.

44 Ibid., vol. 1, p. 275.

45 Jenner to —, 21 September 1803, RCS Box MS0016
4 & 6, Edward Jenner [miscellaneous].

46 Baron, *Life*, vol. 2, pp. 37–8.

47 Ibid., vol. 2, pp. 164–5; Miller, G., *Letters of Edward
Jenner* (Johns Hopkins University Press, 1983),
nos 65, 66.

48 Jenner to Mrs Davies, *c.* 1800, BL Add MS 36540 f. 52.

49 Jenner to Thomas Pruen, n.d., WL MS 5240/47.

50 Jenner to John Clinch, 12 March 1801, RCS
MS0016/2 11.

51 Baron, *Life*, vol. 1, p. 492; Miller, *Letters*, nos 9, 10;
Jenner, G.C., *Evidence at Large*, p. 194; Baron, *Life*,
vol. 1, pp. 513–8.

52 Jenner to Phillips, 16 January 1807, RCP MS 735,
f. 22; Jenner to Alexander Marcet, 30 January 1806,
RSM MSS.514; Baron, *Life*, vol. 2, p. 68; Hansard, HC
Deb., 29 July 1807, first series, vol. 9, cols 1007–15.

53 Royal Jennerian Society Directors' Minutes,
4 December 1802, 16 December 1802, 23 December
1802, WL MS 4302.

54 Royal Jennerian Society Directors' Minutes,
17 March 1807, WL MS 4305.

55 Royal Jennerian Society Directors' Minutes, 3 August 1809, WL MS 4305. See also Jenner to Murray, 1 March 1808, WL MS 5244.

56 Jenner to Pruen, 6 July 1808, WL MS 5240/80.

57 Squirrel's real identity: Baron, *Life*, vol. 2, p. 368; assessment of Birch, Baron, *Life*, vol. 2, p. 382; 'immoveable', Baron, *Life*, vol. 2, p. 29. See Squirrel, R., *Observations Addressed to the Public in General on the Cow-Pox, Showing it to Originate in the Scrophula* (W. Smith, 1805); Birch, J., *Serious Reasons for Uniformly Objecting to the Practice of Vaccination* (J. Smeeton, 1806).

58 Rowley, W., *Cow-Pox Inoculation, No Security Against Small-Pox Infection* (J. Harris, 1805); Cf. Fisher, *Edward Jenner*, p. 164, who gets the chronology wrong.

59 Baron, *Life*, vol. 2, pp. 63–4.

60 Jenner to Dibdin is dated 4 February 1805, Miller, *Letters*, no. 18.

61 Aculeus, *Letters to Dr. Rowley, on his Late Pamphlet, Entitled 'Cow-Pox Inoculation, No Security Against Small-Pox Infection'* (Symonds, 1805), pp. v–vi, also 60.

62 Miller, *Letters*, no. 18; Aculeus, *Letters*, pp. 10, 46.

63 Aculeus, *Letters*, p. v. For Jenner's quoted letter in Thornton's pamphlet see Fisher, *Edward Jenner*, p. 164.

64 Baron, *Life*, vol. 2, p. 64.

65 *Critical Review*, 8 (1806), p. 438; *Anti-Jacobin Review and Magazine*, 24 (1806), p. 326; Hawkins, J.J., 'On

Vaccination', *Philosophical Magazine*, 24 (1806), p. 205; Aculeus, *Letters*, p. 60.

66 Fisher, *Edward Jenner*, p. 164; Aculeus, *Letters*, pp. 36–7, 50–1.

67 Baron, *Life*, vol. 2, p. 383.

68 Ibid., vol. 1, pp. 360–2, 365.

69 Jenner, G.C., *Evidence at Large*, pp. 104–34.

70 Jenner to Marcet, 23 February 1803, RSM MSS.514.

71 See Minutes of the Medical Committee of the Royal Jennerian Society, entries for January to July 1806, WL MS 4304; Royal Jennerian Society Quarterly and Annual Minutes of Court Meetings, WL MS 4303; Jenner to Marcet, 4 August 1806, RSM MSS.514.

72 Royal Jennerian Society Directors' Minutes, 25 February 1808, 17 March 1808, WL MS 4305.

73 Jenner to Marcet, 30 January 1807, 4 July 1809, RSM MSS.514.

74 Jenner to Pruen [1808], WL MS 5240/2; 6 May 1808, WL MS 5240/3.

75 Jenner to Pruen, 26 May 1808, WL MS 5240/4; 9 June 1808, WL MS 5240/5; 11 August 1808, WL MS 5340/6; 6 July 1808, WL MS 5240/80.

76 Jenner to Pruen, 2 September 1808, WL MS 5240/8; 14 September 1808, WL MS 5240/9; 23 October 1808, WL MS 5240/10; 21 November 1808, WL 5240/11.

77 Baron, *Life*, vol. 2, p. 120.

78 Jenner to Pruen, 9 January 1809, WL MS 5240/14.

79 Baron, *Life*, vol. 2, p. 124.

80 Jenner to Pruen, 9 January 1809, WL MS 5240/14.

81 Jenner to Pruen, 6 March 1809, WL MS 5240/19.

82 Jenner to John King, 11 June 1809, WL MS 5236; Jenner to Murray, 30 June 1813, WL MS 5245.

83 Jenner to Gardner, 23 October 1821, RCS MS0016/2 34. For the memorandum, or 'circular letter', see Baron, *Life*, vol. 2, pp. 272–3. It appeared as 'Letter Addressed to the Medical Profession Generally, Relative to Vaccination', *London Medical and Physical Journal*, 45 (1821), pp. 277–80.

84 Jenner to Pruen, 27 June 1816, WL MS 5240/61.

85 Baron, *Life*, vol. 1, p. 101.

86 Baron, *Life*, vol. 2, p. 5.

87 RCP MS736, Regulations and Transaction of the Glocestershire [*sic*] Medical Society Instituted May 1788, 28 July 1790.

88 Baron, J., *Illustrations of the Enquiry Respecting Tuberculous Diseases* (Greenwood, 1822).

89 RCP MS372, Edward Jenner Diary, n.d.

90 RCP MS372, Edward Jenner Diary, 20 March 1796; 15 March 1796.

91 RCP MS372, Edward Jenner Diary, n.d.

92 Fosbroke, *Berkeley Manuscripts*, pp. 236–7.

93 Jenner to Astley Cooper, n.d., RCS MS0016/2 22.

94 Jenner to Pruen, 21 November 1808, WL MS 5240/11; Miller, *Letters*, no. 48.

95 Jenner to Pruen, [1809], WL MS 5240/25, see also Miller, *Letters*, no. 46; Jenner to Pruen, [1809], WL MS 5240/28.

96 Miller, *Letters*, no. 49; Jenner to Pruen, 14 February 1810, WL MS 5240/31; Baron, *Life*, vol. 2, pp. 141–2.

97 Jenner to Pruen, 23 October 1815, WL MS 5240/59; Baron, *Life*, vol. 2, p. 219.

98 Ibid., vol. 2, p. 221; Miller, *Letters*, no. 76; Jenner to Pruen, 2 January 1816, WL MS 5240/60; 27 June 1816, WL MS 5240/61.

99 Baron, *Life*, vol. 2, p. 304.

100 Jenner to Pruen, April 1817, WL MS 5240/63; Jenner to Edward Davies, 2 March 1821, WL MS 5237/1.

101 Baron, *Life*, vol. 2, pp. 308–9.

102 Miller, *Letters*, nos 90, 95; Baron, *Life*, vol. 2, pp. 309–10; Jenner to Baron, 31 May 1821, RCS MS0016/2 33; Baron, *Life*, vol. 2, p. 314.

103 Thomas Jefferson to Jenner (via G.C. Jenner), 14 May 1806, in Baron, *Life*, vol. 2, pp. 94–5.

104 Empson, J., 'Little Honoured in his own Country: Statues in Recognition of Edward Jenner MD FRS', *Journal of the Royal Society of Medicine*, 89 (1996), pp. 514–18; Baron, *Life*, vol. 2, pp. 319–20.

105 Hansard, HC Deb, 10 May 1858, third series, vol. 150, col. 354.

106 Vaccination Act, 3 & 4 Vict. c. 29, 1840.

107 Vaccination Act, 16 & 17 Vict. c. 100, 1853.

108 Lambert, R.J., 'A Victorian National Health Service: State Vaccination 1855–71', *Historical Journal*, 5 (1962), pp. 1–18.

109 Durbach, N., *Bodily Matters: The Anti-Vaccination Movement in England, 1853–1907* (Duke University Press, 2005).

110 Darwin, C., *Life of Erasmus Darwin*, ed. Desmond King-Hele (Cambridge University Press, 2003), p. 83.

111 Wallace, A.R., *Vaccination a Delusion: Its Penal Enforcement a Crime* (Swan Sonnenschein, 1898).

112 Scally, G, 'Leave Jenner in Peace: Response to Gareth Williams, "Put Edward Jenner's Statue Back in Trafalgar Square"', *British Medical Journal*, 340 (2010), c. 1980.

113 Fenner, F., Henderson, D.A., Arita, I., Ježek, Z., Ladnyi, I.D., *Smallpox and its Eradication* (World Health Organization, 1988).

114 Jenner, G.C., *Evidence at Large*, p. 7.

115 Thomas Jefferson to Jenner (via G.C. Jenner), 14 May 1806, in Baron, *Life*, vol. 2, pp. 94–5.

116 Williams, G., "Put Edward Jenner's Statue Back in Trafalgar Square"', *British Medical Journal*, 340 (2010), c. 1582.

Further Reading

Bazin, Hervé, *The Eradication of Smallpox: Edward Jenner and The First and Only Eradication of a Human Infectious Disease* (London: Academic Press, 2000)

Brunton, Deborah, *The Politics of Vaccination: Practice and Policy in England, Wales, Ireland, and Scotland, 1800-1874* (Rochester, N.Y.: University of Rochester Press, 2008)

Durbach, Nadja, *Bodily Matters: The Anti-Vaccination Movement in England, 1853–1907* (Durham: Duke University Press, 2005)

Fisher, Richard B., *Edward Jenner: A Biography* (London: Andre Deutsch, 1991)

Hopkins, Donald R., *The Greatest Killer: Smallpox in History* (Chicago: The University of Chicago Press, 1983)

Koplow, David A., *Smallpox: The Fight to Eradicate a Global Scourge* (Berkeley: University of California Press, 2003)

Porter, Dorothy and Roy Porter, 'The Politics of Anti-vaccinationism and Public Health in Nineteenth-century England', *Medical History*, 32 (1988): 231–52

Lambert, R.J., 'A Victorian National Health Service: State Vaccination 1855–71', *Historical Journal*, 5 (1962): 1–18

Moynell, Elinor, 'French Reactions to Jenner's Discovery of Smallpox Vaccination: The Primary Sources', *Social History of Medicine* 8 (1995): 285–303

Miller, Genevieve, *The Adoption of Inoculation for Smallpox in England and France* (Philadelphia: University of Pennsylvania Press, 1957)

Moore, James, *The History of the Small Pox* (London: Longman, 1815)

Tucker, Jonathan B., *Scourge: The Once and Future Threat of Smallpox* (New York: Grove Press, 2001)

Williams, Gareth, *Angel of Death: The Story of Small Pox* (Houndmills: Palgrave Macmillan, 2010)

Williamson, Stanley, *The Vaccination Controversy: The Rise, Reign and Fall of Compulsory Vaccination for Smallpox* (Liverpool: Liverpool University Press, 2007)

Web Links

Dr Jenner's House
www.jennermuseum.com

Hunterian Museum
www.rcseng.ac.uk/museums-and-archives/hunterian-museum

Royal College of Physicians
www.rcplondon.ac.uk/resources/library

Royal College of Surgeons of England
www.rcseng.ac.uk/library

Royal Society of Medicine
www.rsm.ac.uk/library.aspx

The History of Vaccines
www.historyofvaccines.org

The Jenner Institute
www.jenner.ac.uk

Wellcome Library Archives and Manuscripts:
wellcomelibrary.org/collections/about-the-collections/archives-and-manuscripts

Acknowledgements

Thanks to Tony Morris for the inspiration to write this book, to Stephanie Olsen, Michèle Cohen, Greg Fisher, Michele Haapamäki and Martin Lücke for bearing witness to the research, and to the following for making the research possible: The Royal College of Surgeons of England; The Royal College of Physicians of England; The Royal Society of Medicine; The British Library; The Wellcome Library, London; the Deutsche Forschungsgemeinschaft and the Center for the History of Emotions, Max Planck Institute for Human Development.

About the Author

Rob Boddice (PhD, FRHistS) is Senior Research Fellow at the Academy of Finland Centre of Excellence in the History of Experiences. He is the author/editor of thirteen books, including *Knowing Pain: A History of Sensation, Emotion and Experience* (Polity Press, 2023), *Humane Professions: The Defence of Experimental Medicine, 1876–1914* (Cambridge University Press, 2021) and *A History of Feelings* (Reaktion, 2019).